The Power of Rolfing (SI)

What Rolfing Structural Integration Can Do for You

Owen Marcus

Published in the United States by New Tribe Press
ISBN: 978-0-9887035-1-3

The Power of Rolfing (SI)
What Rolfing Structural Integration
Can Do for You

Table of Contents

The Secrets of the Science and Art of Rolfing® SI

Introduction

The goal of this e-book is to give you a quick and simple guide to Rolfing® Structural Integration (SI), what it might do for you, and how it works. Or for those who want a friend or family member to experience the benefits of Rolfing® (SI).

Much of the content in this e-book was adapted from articles I wrote for several publications as part of the Sandpoint Wellness Council (in Sandpoint, ID). As a reader of this book, you are one of the many people looking for new solutions to your problems. As local healthcare providers, we formed the Wellness Council to give people the knowledge they need to make new choices and find those solutions.

For more than 60 years, people have continued to seek out Rolfing® SI to fix or enhance what other therapies can't. After 30 plus years of practice and more than one thousand clients, I have not only learned more about Rolfing® SI, but I have learned how to explain it and describe the unique benefits it offers people. This therapy with a strange name is actually easy to understand.

The first part of this book describes in clear terms the science and art of Rolfing® SI. The second part discusses many of the conditions that Rolfing® SI has successfully helped to treat. The last part of the book explains the effects Rolfing® SI has on clients.

Please use this book as a guide to explore what Rolfing® SI may do for you or your friends, and share it with others.

For more information on Rolfing® SI, to locate a qualified Certified Rolfer™, to learn how to become a Certified Rolfer™, and for the latest research on Rolfing® SI and fascia (fascia is the connective tissue Certified Rolfers™ release), visit the website of the Rolf institute: www.rolf.org.

Overview of Rolfing® SI

I am the first to admit that naming a technique Rolfing was not the best marketing move. Ida Rolf, Ph.D., the founder, would have agreed. It wasn't her choice...the name just stuck.

If you are like most people, you have heard a few things about Rolfing® Structural Integration (SI). You may have heard it hurts. Yes, there can be some pain, much like getting in shape or stretching can be painful (more on this later). But Rolfing® SI still exists after 60 years and more than a million clients because it works. It is not a panacea, but if stress relief, soft tissue repair, or structure realignment are your issues or goals, Rolfing® may be the best thing for you.

The Four Reasons to Experience Rolfing® SI

Fix the Unfixable

Many of the clients who find their way to a Certified Rolfer's™ door do so because she or he has "tried everything." These people want to be well and have often invested tens of thousands of dollars to discover what is wrong and how to fix it. They might have tried surgery, medication, physical therapy, chiropractic...and yet the pain remains. After a multitude of tests, nothing shows up. Some are labeled hypochondriacs or are relegated to taking psychotropic drugs to treat their "emotional problems."

When medical tests don't find the cause of a problem, holistic health therapies can often go beyond finding the diagnosis to helping the client heal it. Rolfing® SI is particularly good at treating chronic soft tissue problems, such as tight muscles and stress-related issues like hypertension. As we get older we accumulate more tension in our bodies. This stress and tension ends up in the fascia[1] (the connective tissue of our body that holds everything together).

---

[1] http://en.wikipedia.org/wiki/Fascia

There is no medical test for the relative buildup of fascial tension. There is no drug or physical therapy to release that stress. Over time, this tension pulls on your bones, your joints, and your internal organs. Rolfers™ abilities to identify and then release chronic and acute tension set us apart from other professions. When I had my clinic in Scottsdale, AZ, physicians would send me patients to determine why the standard therapies weren't working. Often it was because the real cause of the problem was not actually located anywhere near where the symptom had presented itself. Particularly with chronic problems, the fascial network will tighten in one area only to manifest a problem in another.

For most patients, until the chronic tension is released, no lasting improvement is possible. One of the goals of Rolfing® is to release the chronic tension of the body, freeing the body to heal itself.

Improve Performance

A tight body is not only more prone to injury and pain; its performance is limited. It is as if you're attempting to move in a jumpsuit that is too small. Part of the problem is that the jumpsuit gradually shrinks over many years causing you to lose awareness of its effect on your performance. All of this is compounded by dysfunction caused by past injuries, compensatory patterns, and the fact that your shrinking jumpsuit creates imbalances across joints (some areas becoming too long or lax).

As Certified Rolfers ™ we began speaking about core muscles back in the 1960s, and people thought we were nuts. Now with the growth of Pilates and yoga, core strength is a hot topic, and rightfully so. When your movement and power comes from those deep muscles you are less likely to injure yourself and more likely to perform better. Frequently people are so bound up that even with good instruction they are unable to fully access their core. Some will just end up making their core muscles tighter as they get stronger.

With Rolfing® SI, a client will not only release the chronic stress, they'll also be able to access their core muscles and learn to use gravity as their ally. True core usage and natural use of gravity go together. From my experience working with elite athletes, I learned that this relationship was frequently the difference between winning and losing.

Improve Quality of Life

Most clients come to Rolfing® SI to relieve pain. So why do they return when, after just a few sessions, the pain is often gone? They come back for the subtle benefits of feeling better. With their chronic stress and old traumas leaving, clients' bodies begin to feel young. What might have seemed like an emotional block just melts away with the release of tension in your body.

Learning to breathe naturally and relax is significant. These benefits may not be understood until the tension leaves. When the tight jumpsuit is removed, you are free.

The Best Investment

Numerous times over the years, I have heard clients say that the severe physical pain that drove them to Rolfing® SI was the best thing that could have happened to them. It was the pain that got them to try something as strange as Rolfing® SI, which gave them their body back.

We often behave like a frog in water that is slowly coming to a boil. The pain develops so gradually that we don't think to jump out until well past the point of comfort. Once out of the boiling water, we ask "Why did I wait so long?" Until we feel better, we don't know what we were missing. An investment in Rolfing® SI has the ability not only to remove the pain, but also to prevent future problems from developing. You'll never get caught in boiling water again!

After the series of Rolfing® SI sessions, clients will report that resolving their initial complaint wasn't the largest benefit; it was feeling alive again.

Common Benefits

Note: this is not a guarantee, but here are some examples to give you a sense of what is possible. Certified Rolfers™ frequently see these benefits in clients.

- Chronic stress and pain reduction

- Injury prevention and recovery

- Improved athletic performance

- Improved stamina

- Improved posture and gait

- Healthier appearance

- Healing of post traumatic stress disorder (PTSD)

- Weight lost and cellulite reduction

- Enhanced circulation

- Improved digestive and organ function

- Chronic fatigue release and healing

- Fibromyalgia healing

- Healing and prevention of repetitive motion injuries

- Increased flexibility and coordination

- Chronic headaches disappearing

- Back pain healing

- TMJ pain elimination

- Emotional stress transforming into relaxation

- More vital energy

- Enhanced wellbeing

- Improved relaxation and sleep

- Greater enjoyment of the body

What Rolfing® SI Is Best at Treating?

If your problems or goals fall into any of these categories, Rolfing® SI may be beneficial for you.

Structure

What most will call posture, Certified Rolfers™ call structure. Posture is the behavioral consequence of structure. Your body's structural order will determine how you move.

To start with, most of what we were told was good posture—shoulders back, chest up, and stomach in—are more indicative of a stress response than good posture. Good posture is effortless. Many of the muscles we use to stand and move were not designed for those functions. When a muscle, or for that matter any body part, repeatedly does a job it is not designed to do, it produces stress and tension.

If you want to be straight and move with grace, find a Certified Rolfer™. By releasing the chronic tension, and with a little coaching, you can learn to significantly improve your appearance and movement.

Soft Tissue

Soft tissue is exactly what it sounds like: it is the muscles and the fascia—the connective tissue that contains all our body parts. Hans Selye, MD, published his book, *The Stress of Life* in 1956, calling fascia the organ of stress. When physical or emotional stress is not released, it is stored in the fascial network throughout the body, reproducing stress even when the stressor is gone. You feel it as soft tissue tightens up.

There is no drug or surgery that releases that type of tension. In holistic health treatments, there are several techniques, such as acupuncture and massage that do a great job of releasing more acute tension. Rolfing® SI excels at releasing chronic tension from decades of stress, misuse, and injuries.

Certified Rolfers™ will frequently hear clients say, "I know I would feel better if someone would just loosen me up." Rolfing® SI attempts not only to release the chronic tension, but also prevent it from returning by organizing the body.

Stress

Your fight or flight response (sympathetic nervous system response) is meant to kick in only when you are in danger. Unfortunately, because of the stress in your life, and how you learned to deal with that stress, you may never escape this survival response. Problems arise when you live in a constant state of survival response; the ongoing effect of the response accumulates. The persistent stress response is, in part, perpetuated by tense fascia, which keeps the stress response activated. It is as if your accelerator is stuck, so that your engine revs even when you're in neutral. Just as the car engine will burn out, your body will become old before its time if it continually experiences such stress.

We are beginning to understand the physiology and effects of constant stress through research on Post Traumatic Stress Disorder (PTSD). With PTSD, the stressor might be gone, but the traumatic response continues. Many clients come to Rolfing® SI functioning from some point on the PTSD continuum, experiencing a stress response when there is no stressor.

There is research[2] showing that Rolfing® SI reduces a client's stress response. In layman's terms, that means you can *respond* calmly to stressors, rather than *react* physiologically. Your face doesn't have to flush. Your pulse doesn't need to race. You can simply acknowledge a stressor, and respond to it appropriately.

---

[2] http://rolf.org/about/research.htm#rrr

Where Is Rolfing® SI Best Used?

Rolfing® SI is best used to reduce or eliminate the cause of chronic pain. With the release of chronic tensions, the body can heal itself.

Rolfing® SI is not recommended for those with chronic illnesses involving systemic problems, genetic illnesses, or cancer. If the cause or the effect of the condition does not involve structure, soft tissue, or stress, Rolfing® SI's effectiveness significantly declines.

With some conditions, Rolfing SI® will not affect the disease, but can aid in recovery. Post-polio syndrome is an excellent example of how Rolfing® reverses years of strain from dealing with a disease.

Rolfing® SI's effectiveness in treating chronic conditions does make it effective in treating some acute conditions. Many other therapies, such as massage, chiropractic, and acupuncture, can also treat new problems effectively. It's not that Rolfing® SI can't help that new back tightness, but if that tightness is not built on a tight body, and is truly new and independent of past situations, Rolfing® SI may not be your only solution.

Massage therapy is most effective with acute problems. Physical therapy is best with rehabilitation from injuries and surgeries. Chiropractic treatments are best treating acute problems that cause joints to be out of alignment. A Certified Rolfer's™ focus is on chronic soft tissue problems affecting your structure and your stress response.

Bottom line, if your body needs to release persistent tension and subsequent problems, Rolfing® SI may be the most effective therapy.

How Does Rolfing® SI Work?

Rolfing® SI is a series of progressive, hour-long sessions. Each focuses on particular goals and areas of the body. These goals and areas vary with each client. The Certified Rolfer™ will address your immediate concern as he or she addresses the underlying causes and aligns your body to be in balance with gravity so that the results will have longevity.

The client lies on a wide table in his or her bathing suit, underwear, or workout clothing. The Certified Rolfer™ uses his or her hands, forearms or elbows to release the soft tissue with the goal of bringing more order to the body. Through this sculpting process, the client can experience a deep release of chronic tension.

The Certified Rolfer™ works at the pace of the client's tissue's ability to let go. Enough pressure needs to be used to release the fascial adhesions, but when done slowly and with sensitivity, the pressure is not great.

A Certified Rolfer™ is much like a structural engineer evaluating the structural weaknesses that are not yet presenting problems. The cracks in walls can represent a settling foundation. Until the foundation is repaired, no matter how often the cracks are repaired, they will return. Your body is the same. Until the shortness and rotation in your leg is released, your neck may always be going "out."

The deep changes Rolfing® SI produces will often take up to a year to fully manifest. The tighter your body, the more tension it has. The tension releases at its own pace, one layer at a time. It is common for a client to see more change in six months of integrating the Rolfing® SI changes than from the ten sessions themselves.

The myofascial releases of Rolfing® SI are the foundation for the deep structural realignment and movement enhancements Rolfing® SI is known for creating. Through the release of chronic tension, your nervous system, perception, coordination, and experience of the world can change. A tense body is bracing against the anticipation of future stress. A relaxed body moves out of its way or releases it.

The Release

As you lie on a Rolfing® SI table, your Certified Rolfer™ may lean on her elbow against your thigh. Your first sensation may be pain, producing an urge to resist. Because the Certified Rolfer™ is not increasing her pressure—actually she is just waiting for your tissue to release—you begin to relax. Through relaxing, you surrender to what might have felt like pain, and you start to feel intense sensations. The intensity subsides as the release occurs. With the release increasing, the next sensation is pleasure.

This cycle of intensity to release to pleasure feels much like the one of stretching. The body will learn how to relax much as it does from stretching. The tensions or hypersensitivity that might have first existed can actually feel pleasurable just one session later. You learn to relax and be relaxed. Stimulation (i.e., pressure) goes from something that you want to resist to something that is pleasurable to relax into.

The processes of learning to relax on a deep level will vary with the individual. Tough guys, like myself, will often take longer than women. But you knew that...

Rolf Movement® Integration

Ida Rolf, Ph.D. encouraged the development of movement work to assist Rolfing® clients in their changes and integration. Certified Rolfers™ were always trained in movement work. Recently, all Certified Rolfers™ are being certified as Rolf Movement Practitioners.

Unlearning bad habits and learning more effective ways to use your body can obviously be a huge benefit. Some Certified Rolfers™ integrate Rolfing® Movement Integration in their structural sessions. Others do separate sessions. Either way, being aware of both methods can be very useful. They go beyond ergonomics to learning how to enhance the use of your body through exploring perception and coordination in your everyday movements.

Frequently Asked Questions

Do I have to commit to ten sessions?
No. Most Certified Rolfers™ will just have you pay and schedule as you go. In fact, if for some reason you want to switch Certified Rolfers™ during the series, you can. It is your body and your money.

How often will I have sessions?
Anywhere from twice per week to once a month is the range. Most clients come in once per week. The frequency depends on your body's ability to integrate the work and what works best for you.

Is Rolfing® SI safe?
Yes. As long as you don't have one of the contraindications mentioned earlier (Where Is Rolfing® SI Best Used? Section), it is safe. For a Certified Rolfer™, the goal is not to force change; it is to evoke change through releasing the soft tissue. The soft tissue can't release if the Certified Rolfer™ goes too deep or too fast. Your biggest risk is wasting some time and money.

Is Rolfing® SI just stretching?
No. Rolfing® SI goes beyond stretching or yoga by releasing the tightest and hardest areas of your body. Often in stretching, only the looser places stretch. What needs to stretch are the thick, bound up areas. Stretching often produces frustration, particularly for men with those hard, thick legs. Once Rolfing® SI releases these concrete areas, then stretching can help.

Does Rolfing® SI hurt?
Yes, it can feel painful the first time in very tense areas. It is not the pain of injury. When there is pain, it is from experiencing the tension that was always there. If for some reason, you feel it might be too much, you can tell the Certified Rolfer™ to stop. You are always in charge.

How does Rolfing® SI work with pain?
With chronic pain, clients are often told there is nothing wrong. I have seen clients sent to psychiatrists to treat "imaginary pain." The interesting thing about pain, particularly soft tissue pain, is that there are no definitive tests to evaluate pain.

Chronic pain in itself becomes an escalating condition often only treated with medication. For many, the secret to ending the pain is releasing the tension and training the body to relax. Yes, this sounds simple—sometimes it is that simple. There is an interesting relationship with pain and awareness. The more pain you have, the less awareness you have. The inverse is also true. As you become more aware, which might feel uncomfortable at first, the more you are able to release the tension causing the pain.

A Certified Rolfer™ works to assist you in releasing your chronic tension and pain. They can only do that if you are relaxing. For that to happen, you must first feel safe, then you must feel that you are in control. Only then can you let go of what you might not have been aware of before or had the ability to release.

What age range do Certified Rolfers™ treat?
From infants to the elderly. Most clients are active children or adults.

How does Rolfing® SI affect the aging process?
Through releasing the tension in the fascia, the body becomes more resilient in its structure, movement, and appearance. Most clients report feeling younger because their bodies are behaving as they did when they were young. Much of what we attribute to age is the accumulation of stress and tension.

How does Rolfing® SI affect posttraumatic stress disorder (PTSD), chronic fatigue, fibromyalgia, and depression?
Often a connection between these four debilitating conditions is the physical exhaustion caused by a body being stuck in hyper-arousal or survival mode. Anyone exposed to constant stress will eventually acclimatize to the stress. You learn to adapt emotionally by becoming accustomed to it and by physically sustaining an alert status. No matter how strong you are, eventually the continuous stress will wear you down and may eventually present as one or more of the above conditions.

To heal, your body must first leave the survival state—the revved-up state. Until your body feels safe, it will be allocating its resources to survival. Rolfing® SI has the ability to deeply release the stress and the self-perpetuating survival response stored in the tissue. Once the body comes down, the resources directed to survival can be used for self-healing. Your body can rest and heal.

Owen Marcus

What does the medical community think of Rolfing®?
Physicians are referring their patients to Certified Rolfers™ in increasing numbers for chronic problems. There is a growing understanding and appreciation of Rolfing® SI, in part from Certified Rolfers™ being physicians and many physicians experiencing Rolfing® SI. The growing research on fascia continues to put Rolfing® SI in the spotlight as the therapy that treats fascial conditions.

Does insurance pay for Rolfing® SI?
Auto insurance and workers' comp often pay for Rolfing® SI. Medical insurance is more challenging. A referral from a physician and persistence with your insurance company can increase your chances of being paid.

The growth of consumer-driven healthcare plans (CDHP), wherein the employee and/or employer contribute to a fund pool used to reimburse out-of-pocket expenses for the insurer, creates more options. The funds in plans such as the plans listed below will usually pay for Rolfing® SI.

> FSA — Flexible Spending Account
> MSA — Medical Savings Account
> HRA — Health Reimbursement Arrangement
> HSA — Health Savings Account

What can I expect from a session?
Each session begins by asking you what's happened since the previous session: Is your pain gone? Did you notice anything new? The Certified Rolfer™ will observe how you move and hold your body.

A Rolfing® SI session is not a massage, but like a massage, you will be relaxed afterwards. Clients often report sleeping deeply the night after the first session and feeling relaxed and possibly tired for a few days.

There is usually no soreness after a session. When there is soreness, it isn't the type you get from an injury, but more like the feeling you might have after a good stretch or workout. Do not workout later in the day after receiving a session. The next day should be fine to exercise.

How do I choose a good Certified Rolfer™?

Ask others who have experienced Rolfing® themselves. Check out Certified Rolfers'™ web sites. Call the prospective Certified Rolfer™ personally. Ask him or her all your questions. Trust your gut. Most Certified Rolfers™ will offer a free consultation; if in doubt, try that. You only need to do one session. Yes, it is theoretically possible the Certified Rolfer™ could hurt you. My experience is that it is so rare that there is much greater risk from the effects of your tension seriously impacting your health. The worse thing that is likely to happen is you don't get exactly what you wanted.

Take a risk, give a session a try.

Not all "Rolfers" are Certified Rolfers™

More and more people are claiming they are practicing Rolfing® SI. That's good because it means Rolfing® SI is the go-to therapy. Unfortunately, these other practitioners are not doing Rolfing® SI; they were not trained at the Rolf Institute®. If they are saying "trained in the Rolf method" that is an indication they most likely are not Certified Rolfers™.

Over the years, in most cases when I traced back a complaint about a Certified Rolfer™, the "Rolfer" in question was not a Certified Rolfer™. If you have any doubt, go to the Rolf Institute® web site, www.rolf.org, to verify that the person you are considering is a Certified Rolfer™. The practitioner may be good at what he or she does, but it is not Rolfing® if he or she is not a Certified Rolfer™.

How Rolfing® SI Helps
Common Problems

Here are short explanations of how Rolfing® SI can help some of our most common problems. Realize that everyone is different and there can be other variables at play. In my experience, I continue to see these responses from my clients.

Pain Is An Option

We Love Pain

How is it that the US is only 4.6% of the world population, but we consume 80% of all pain drugs? We are told "no pain, no gain," yet we run to the medicine cabinet for a pain pill at the first sign of discomfort.

Our love of our drugs matches the level of tension in our bodies. Our culture adapted to high stress, but our bodies haven't. Over the years, we become tenser and tenser so slowly and consistently that we are unaware of it. How would you be aware of it when all your friends are responding the same way?

The tensest clients in our clinics are the ones in the most pain. Sure, they had an injury, but what makes it so painful and resistant to standard treatment is the chronic tension. In fact, their tension sets them up for injury – when you're wound really tight, the chances of getting hurt are higher. Then the high stress/tension state inevitably produces a physiology similar to Post Traumatic Stress Disorder (PTSD). The body is in a survival state, orienting all its resources to stay alive.

As you habituate stress and tension, you progressively become less aware of your body. Under stress you don't feel as fully, as if you were running for your life in the forest not feeling the pain of the branches hitting your body. With constant stress, you don't feel the tension build. Then one injury or emotional crisis occurs and you are in serious PAIN. Believing that it was that last incident that caused the pain, you look at treating the immediate problem. The pain is intense because the background chronic tension in your body is significant.

The fear of the pain increases the tension, which increases the pain. You are trapped. Pain drugs may take the edge off, but you run the risk of training your body to where the drugs don't work any longer. All the drug ads telling you a pill will fix it only makes you more stressed. Your doctors want to help, but, as they tell me and a recent *New York Times* article describes, "Drugs are cheaper than a multidisciplinary approach to chronic pain. Doctors get reimbursed to treat people quickly, so funding for other approaches is cut out. These drugs became the treatment method of choice."[3]

Our unrequited love for pain needs to end. We need to understand that we don't need to be a victim to pain or limited by the hope of treating the symptoms through drugs. In the next article, I will speak more about how to escape the pain trap.

What Pain Does

We all know that pain tells us that something is wrong. What we might miss is that the immediate pain is telling us that something was wrong for a while. As we became more stressed and tense, we became less aware. This inverse relationship builds until we have significant pain. When the standard route of treatment is not working and the pain is getting worse, the old coping pattern shifts. It's only when the pain becomes greater than the fear of trying something different that we will muster up the courage to try a new option.

When I had a holistic medical clinic in Scottsdale, AZ, we operated the largest Mindfulness Based Stress Reduction program in the country. Hospitals and corporations would send us their chronic pain patients and stressed-out people. These students were the people others gave

---

[3] New York Times, *The Problem With Pain Pills*, June 26, 2013

up on helping. Through eight weeks of 45 minutes of practice per day plus a weekly class, we were continually amazed at how the students transformed. Chronic pain students would be off their pain meds and suffering no pain within weeks.

What we were teaching couldn't have been simpler. We were teaching the students to do the opposite of what they'd perfected: rather than attempt not to feel their bodies or their pain—or tighten up against it— we taught them to feel. As they felt and breathed, they relaxed. As they relaxed, a little of their tension would release. At first, these small acts of surrendering were scary. It was going against everything we all were trained to do.

We had athletes, physicians, and corporate executives coming in each week sharing their stories of how their pain was gone, how they weren't stressed out, and how they were getting more done. They realized that their chronic pain was more a function of their chronic stress conditioning than that last accident. Just like in my Rolfing® SI practice, once people have a little improvement from some non-standard approach, they are fully committed to doing what it takes to get rid of all the pain.

No one wants to be in pain. Most people have the smarts and courage to do what it takes to get out of pain. Understandably, after the experience of many drugs, treatments, and shelling out of money, these people were hesitant to try "another treatment." One thing chronic pain does is wear you out—you become discouraged. When others tell you there is nothing that can be done, it's understandable that you're depressed.

Many years ago, a woman sent her friend to me for Rolfing® SI. The client sat on my couch describing how at the end of the week at the Mayo Clinic, the best that they could suggest was the woman see their psychiatrist. When I walked over to touch the places I saw that were tense and in pain, she began crying. In her tears, she said, "You're the first person who believed me."

A New Model

Andrew Weil, MD, the Harvard-trained holistic physician, would say in our planning meetings, allopathic medicine is not set up to treat chronic illness. Chronic means it existed for some time. It's not a tibia you broke skiing, it's that back pain that won't go away.

"There are plenty of data suggesting that a multidisciplinary approach to chronic pain works as effectively as high-dose opioid treatment…. What insurers and workers' comp agencies are discovering is that when workers are treated with high doses of opioid drugs fairly soon after these injuries, it's the leading predictor for them not coming back to work for long periods of time, or ever. "[4]

Most people want more than to "treat" their pain. They want to eliminate it. This is possible with the release of the cause of the pain. The pain represents the tip of the iceberg of an old problem. The iceberg needs melting. As the previous article described, going from fighting the pain to accepting the body sensations, then to releasing the resistance can be transformational.

After 35 years and more than a thousand clients, my biggest realization is that when the body releases its tension all the resources that went into what the body experienced as survival can be allocated to healing. If a mountain lion is chasing you, you will do everything to escape. You won't feel the pain of running into branches. Surviving depends on using every ounce of energy to run for your life. This is what chronic pain does to you. You are trying to survive.

Getting your autonomic nervous system to shift from the sympathetic state (the survival state) to the parasympathetic state (the rejuvenation state) is the key to addressing the cause of most chronic pain. Your body's soft tissue system is your stress holder. Much like a rubber band

---

[4] New York Times, *The Problem With Pain Pills*, June 26, 2013

wound tight, your tight body is holding a lot of stored tension—which is the classic set up for pain.

The older or worse the chronic pain, the more chronic tension in the body, which means the more you release that tension, the less pain you will have. There is no drug that will cause your body to release tension, there are those, including alcohol, that will mask the tension. To attain the depth of relaxation to release the pain, you need to do more than "relax." After years of tension, your body lost its ability to relax on its own.

Mindfulness Based Stress Reduction retrains your body and mind the forgotten skill of relaxation. Deeper massage over time will release and retrain the body as will yoga. As will other forms of soft tissue manipulation such as visceral manipulation, Rolfing® SI, and possibly acupuncture. As a Rolfer, I tend to be the last resort for the super tense. When other therapies can't get a hard body to relax, the practitioners send the patients to a Rolfer. I say that with a little dread, because it's hard work working on a tense body—until they let go. I know this from having super tense clients, but also from being one myself.

How to Heal Repetitive Injuries

Repetitive strain injuries cost the nation more than $20 billion a year. The average cost per workman's compensation claim exceeds $12,000. And these repetitive strain (or motion) injuries are getting worse. Repetitive micro-traumas cause inflammation in the soft tissue.[5] They cause scarring and impinge upon nerves, leading to devastating pain. Many people suffering from micro-traumas try physical therapy, drugs, surgery, or other solutions only to have the pain persist.

Often these people don't even realize what's truly causing their chronic pain.[6] Their posture, movement patterns and body tension are perpetuating the problem. Fixing the symptom often doesn't last because the cause lies in other areas of the body.

Healing the Cause of Repetitive Injuries

Once you step back to look at why a particular part of the body continues to be painful or injured, you see how that body part's movement is not performing according to its intended design. Your body is very adaptive, but if you must repeat a particular movement, it needs to be done in the most efficient manner. Efficient body mechanics require a relaxed and aligned body.

As you get older, your body is less resilient not because of aging, but because of increased systemic tension and declining alignment. Eventually, your weak links break. I've seen runners' chronic knee injuries return after multiple successful surgeries because the misaligned leg remained. I've seen professional baseball pitchers' rotator cuff injuries[7] return because the shoulder was attempting to compensate for misaligned legs.

---

[5] http://en.wikipedia.org/wiki/Soft_tissue

[6] http://en.wikipedia.org/wiki/Chronic_pain

[7] http://www.mayoclinic.com/health/rotator-cuff-injury/DS00192/

Think of your chronic injury, usually around a joint, as being the misaligned wheel. You could keep replacing the unevenly worn tire, or you can realign the wheel. Any mechanical device will wear out before its time if the stress placed on the part is inappropriate.

Through 2.5 million years of refinement, our structures have developed effective ways to do repetitive tasks. If they hadn't, we wouldn't be here today. Our ancestors first hunted by outrunning their prey (see persistence hunting). If they were injured, they starved.

What You Can Do for Your Repetitive Injuries

Find a Rolfer® who works with natural alignment, soft tissue release, and natural movement patterns. I emphasize *natural* because most of our posture cues are handed down unquestioned. For example, standing aligned does not mean holding your shoulders back. You need someone who helps you release the underlying cause of your tension while helping you unlearn ineffective movement patterns. Rolfing® SI is a proven therapy to help repetitive motion/strain injuries.

Solving Foot Problems

Is there anything about your feet that just doesn't work? Do you have one of these common feet conditions:

- plantar fasciitis[8] (tightness and pain in the bottom of the foot)
- heel spurs (bone growth due to strain)
- neuromas (pinched nerve)
- bunions (the big toe is bent)

---

[8] http://en.wikipedia.org/wiki/Plantar_fasciitis

The Problem

Whatever your problem, it is likely it is caused by:

- improper walking
- structural misalignment
- soft tissue tension

You might say, "I inherited this condition. It's genetics." But your soft tissue tension, movement patterns, and much of your structure are not just genetic, but they are learned at an early age. Sometimes, you learned it so early and so unconsciously it seems genetic.

When any part of your body experiences constant strain, even slight strain, that part will create scar tissue over time to protect and heal the area. For example, a high arch often creates more strain for the plantar fascia, the connective tissue on the bottom of the foot. Eventually this fascial irritation becomes painful as each step strains it further. For some people the standard remedies, such as orthotics, may help for a while. For others, the only permanent remedy is releasing the fascia of the whole leg, not just the foot. The stride of the whole leg affects how the foot lands, so the problem will return if the stride is not changed.

The Solution

The 26 bones of the feet sit in a soft tissue sock. The tendons act like a puppeteer's strings, traveling up to the muscles of the lower leg. The sock gets tight and distorted, but often much of the problem comes from above the foot. For example, the posterior tibialis muscle[9] along with its tendon is part of the stirrup that lifts the arch. All babies start with flat feet. How you develop your walk determines how your arch develops. If you're flat-footed like me, your walk developed as the result of misuse of the posterior tibialis, which caused it to become tight. I was amazed to see my flat feet change back in the 70's when I experi-

---

[9] http://en.wikipedia.org/wiki/Tibialis_anterior_muscle

enced Rolfing® SI. They're still somewhat flat, but they are less so. Most importantly, they work well now.

While in Scottsdale, I treated many runners. Once we released the tension and aligned their legs and feet, I went on to teach them the *Natural Walk* (which is the basis for the run) and their problems disappeared. In every case, these runners ran faster.

What to Do When Orthotics Don't Work

If you are one of the thousands of people who support the $5 billion-a-year industry of orthotics, there is a good chance you are frustrated because they aren't working. A *New York Times* article asked Benno M. Nigg, a professor of biomechanics at the University of Calgary, whether orthotics work. His reply: "The idea that they are supposed to correct mechanical-alignment problems does not hold up." Even a leading podiatrist blog questions orthotics usefulness.

What Orthotics Do

Orthotics act as a shim to adjust for a leg-length discrepancy or for an imbalance in the foot, such as flat feet. Most orthotics, particularly the expensive ones made by podiatrists, are hard plastic. We have 26 bones in each foot because the foot is meant to move. As explained by the research barefoot runner[10] enthusiasts often quote, the more "support" a shoe or orthotic gives, the worse the injuries are.

When I had my clinic in Scottsdale we treated hundreds of runners. Some were Olympic middle- and long-distance runners. All of the runners—yes, ALL—who came in with orthotics got rid of them. They learned to walk and run in such a way that they no longer needed expensive orthotics, AND their injuries went away and their running improved.

---

[10] http://en.wikipedia.org/wiki/Barefoot_running

After several pairs of orthotics, a runner learns that all orthotics do is shift the strain to another part of the body. For a while some runners saw improvements, but inevitably, the injury would return or an injury would develop somewhere else, such as in their legs, hip, or back.

What Can Work

My approach is to start with the least invasive and least expensive approach: change your stride. Barefoot running works for so many people because it forces them to change their stride so that it matches the way our bodies are designed to move, allowing the legs and feet to move as they are meant to move. With each stride the foot bends, stretches, and subtly flexes. When a person changes his stride, in most cases, whatever imbalance caused him to try orthotics is gone. (See the section on Natural Walking™ and Natural Running™ for further explanation.)

You could go barefoot. More runners and clients of mine are doing it—and every single person with whom I've spoken about barefoot running won't go back. That says something.

Good stretching or yoga can help, as can specific massage designed to release the soft tissue—but these therapies don't release the deeper more chronic tension, nor do they realign the body. Here's an insider tip: tightness in the foot is not only in the foot... it's in the lower leg. That's where the major muscles for the foot reside. The foot itself gets tight from the fascia of the foot getting tight, which causes plantar fasciitis. But fixing the foot always involves releasing and organizing the lower leg.

When the soft tissue is released and realigned, not only in the feet and legs, but in the whole body, the feet stop taking the hit—and they stop hurting.

Roll Your Troubles Away

Certainly for us guys, stretching the way we were taught is not fun or even productive. Men often come to me because they go to a yoga class and realize how tight they really are. Lying on a rubber mat next to a young woman rapping her legs around her neck when you can't even sit on the floor with your legs crossed is more than embarrassing. It's humbling.

I cheated. I got Rolfed when I was in my early 20s. In the course of 10 sessions and the subsequent nine months of my body letting go, I went from a body of solid gristle to being able to sit on the floor with my legs fully crossed and knees flat on the floor--my fascia, the connective tissue that becomes scar tissue and gristle, had become supple for the first time in my life.

A foam roller isn't Rolfing® SI, but it isn't stretching either. Akin to Rolfing® SI, it creates a release, which is different than a stretch. Look at this way: you can't stretch a steel cable as if it's a bungee cord. To take the deep adhesions out of the fascia, you need to release the hydrogen bonds that act as the dried glue making the tissue non-resilient. The edge of my arm does that for my Rolfing® SI clients. The edge of a hard foam roller does it for others.

Using your own gravity, you allow yourself to slowly relax your weight on to the roller. For best results you aren't rolling, you are melting. Rolling on hard tissue is just like rubbing it. We know that's not going to release the deeper and harder tissue. You need to go slow so the deeper adhesions release. More yoga studios here in Sandpoint are incorporating foam rollers in their classes.

The outside of the upper leg, the Iliotibial band, is usually the hardest and tightest part of our bodies. Rolling this band can be much more effective than stretching. Unfortunately I have seen men who were too tight for rolling to be effective--I was one of them. In that case it takes someone who knows what they are doing to get the process started. When I Rolfed elite runners in Arizona, I found once we got their legs to loosen and straighten, rolling was all they needed for maintenance.

You Want to Be Smarter, Happier and Sexier— Feed Your Bones

New research is showing us that our bones do much more than just hold up our skin. They nourish us, and communicate to other parts of our body. Bones are part of the connective tissue system that includes the blood, fascia, tendons, ligaments, and cartilage. Jim Oshman, an old friend of mine and a scientist for NIH, proved decades ago that the acupuncture points are connected to specific organs through the fascia system. Now Gerard Karsenty, chair of the Department of Genetics and Development at Columbia University Medical Center is showing that our bones are more than just the framework for our muscles.

In a recent *New Yorker* article, Karsenty explains:

> The finding represents new ground in how researchers view the skeleton: not only do bones provide structural support and serve as a repository for calcium and phosphate, they issue commands to far-flung cells. In mice at least, they talk directly to the brain. "This is a biggie," said Eric Kandel, the neuroscientist and Nobel Laureate. "Who thinks of the bone as being an endocrine organ? You think of the adrenal gland, you think of the pituitary, you don't think of bone.[11]

It seems that the protein osteocalcin is a messenger, like a hormone sent by bones to regulate essential processes all over the body. Ostecalcin has been proven to have "effects on mice's fat stores, livers, muscles, pancreases, testes, and even, as new evidence suggests, their brains."[12]

The article goes on to explain how our bones can be linked to memory loss, anxiety, depression and male reproduction for mice. As we age, we

---

[11] "Do Our Bones Influence Our Minds? : The New Yorker," November 4, 2013.

[12] Ibid.

need to keep our bones strong, and not just to prevent osteoporosis; our bones need to be strong if we are to remain vital.

The research done with Super Slow training shows how just fifteen minutes of slow resistance per week can dramatically turn around osteoporosis. The anecdotal evidence supports that this form of resistance training can improve an older client's general well-being.

Our bones need more than calcium to function. They need animal protein to help rebuild. The popularity of shark fin soup in China for just that purpose is a huge reason sharks have become an endangered species. You can get the same benefit from making bone broth soup. As with all connective tissue, bones grow according to the stress placed on them; without regular resistance they will deteriorate. So, suck on your soup bones and get out and exercise.

Fat, the Final Frontier

We can carry on a video phone call with anyone on the planet, but we can't win our war on fat. An obese person in America is likely to incur $1,450 in medical expenses annually; we are in crisis. It's true, we're getting smarter – we're realizing what we were told about diet was wrong. It's not fat that makes you fat; it's all the sugar that puts on the pounds.

When I had my clinic in Scottsdale, I had a line of women come to see me to lose cellulite. I never promoted this benefit of Rolfing® SI. It was women noticing the change in their friends. These women lost their hips because most of them were protein deficient, so when they started eating more meat, they toned up. The other factor was releasing the chronic, deep tension that prevents circulation from reaching the cellulite tissue, causing a detoxing inefficiency.

Then there are those who are obsessed with being thin. Our ancestors used their body fat as their reserve for lean times. To this end, a recent study showed that women with bigger butts are smarter and more resistant to disease.[13]

Next to carbohydrate intake, stress is a determiner of your fat. If your body is constantly under stress, you are telling your body's physiology that you are in a state of survival. That causes disruption in your hormones. Your cortisol goes up as your fat goes up. Men will report low testosterone and high estrogen, which is a set up for the most dangerous fat – visceral fat.[14]

Overweight men report low testosterone associated with obesity and sexual dysfunction, along with cardiovascular disease risk and Type 2 diabetes.

Simple Solutions

When clients reduce or eliminate their wheat intake, move more, start breathing properly (most of us breathe a fraction of what is possible), and remove their chronic tension, fat dropped off magically. You don't need to diet; you need to eat well. With sitting becoming the new smoking, most of us don't move enough, let alone exercise enough. Lack of the good stress of movement and exercise has the body tighten and stagnate. Research shows that a good walk is almost as beneficial as a run for exercise.

---

[13] "Women With Big Butts Are Smarter And Resistant To Chronic Illnesses," University Herald, Oct 31, 2013

[14] Low testosterone associated with obesity and the metabolic syndrome contributes to sexual dysfunction and cardiovascular disease risk in men with Type 2 diabetes, PubMed, Jul 2013

Do You Wear Flip Flops?

Of course you do. Everybody does. They're cheap, they're convenient, they are *the* summer footwear—and they have been for decades. Flip flops evolved from the traditional woven-soled Japanese zori used as beach wear in New Zealand in the 1930s. These sandals came to the US with our returning WWII troops.

Unfortunately, they make you more vulnerable to injuries, and produce long-term problems.

Why Wearing Flip Flops Isn't Good

When you walk in flip flops—or any shoe that has no heel strap—you automatically adjust your stride and how you use your foot to keep the sandals on. Whether they're $1.99 flip flops from the grocery store or $100 Birkenstocks, you will walk right out of them if you don't adjust your step. Watch others walk around in them and you'll start to see what I mean. Try it yourself. Put on a pair and walk like you were walking barefoot. Better yet, run in them. It is virtually impossible. A man running in flip flops looks like a woman running in high heels: their heels never touch the ground.

In 2008, Auburn University researchers found that wearing flip-flops can cause sore feet, ankles, and legs. The research showed flip-flop wearers took shorter steps. This stride produced problems from the foot to the hips. During the seventeen years at my clinic in Arizona, I saw many clients who had feet, ankle, knee, hip, and even back problems caused, in part, by the flip-flop stride. Long-time flip-flop wearers have thick and tense lower calves from years of never stretching them out with a natural stride. If you want a shapely leg, don't wear these sandals.

Solutions

If you don't want tense feet and calves, change your shoes. If you don't want to go barefoot, you can simply find a sandal that has a heel strap. They may not be as cool, cheap, or easy to put on as a flip flop, but your body will appreciate it.

Many people are re-discovering walking or running naturally through barefoot running.[15] Moving around barefoot, or in some of the new "barefoot shoes," can slowly release the tension built up by shoes that originally created unnatural stride and structural adjustments.

Do Your Knees Need Help?

The Problem

When you go for a run, ski down a mountain, or go for a bike ride, do your knees hurt? A lot of people think, "I'm getting old," or, "My knee has never been the same since that injury." But it could be a simple problem of misalignment. My experience with hundreds of clients with knee problems has shown me that the vast majority of these problems start as a misalignment.

When they move as they were designed to move, your knees are strong joints. But if the lower leg (tibia) and the upper leg (femur) are not moving parallel to each other, the torque goes to the knee joint, the weak link in the leg. A knee is a "hinge joint," just like a door hinge. When it doesn't move straight, the uneven strain gradually produces pain.

A misaligned wheel produces uneven wear on a tire, and a misaligned leg produces uneven wear, usually at the knee. The question is...where is the imbalance? Sometimes, the foot/ankle complex can be out of balance, producing strain in the leg. Orthotics for a foot problem can cause a knee problem through misalignment. Many of the runners I have treated complained that their knee problem began when they got their new pair of orthotics.

Most frequently though, the main strain is in the upper leg and/or the pelvis (hip). Specifically, the IT band (iliotibial band of fascia on the out-

---

[15] http://en.wikipedia.org/wiki/Barefoot_running

side of the upper leg) becomes very tight, shortening as it twists, pulling unevenly on the knee.

Wherever the misalignment is, over time the repetitive motion of the knee joint produces a strain, then pain. Generally, the strain and pain start on the outside of the knee. If the misalignment continues, the meniscus (knee cartilage) can wear.

The Solution

As a Certified Rolfer™, I see the bones sitting in a system of soft tissue that has shortened, hardened, and twisted. Unevenly pulled strings on a puppet will create a tangled mess, right? Well, imbalances of the 650+ skeletal muscles in your body will pull your bones out of place. Before any significant or sustainable improvement can be made, the imbalances need to be aligned. Releasing your knee will not hold if the strain keeps pulling on it.

Once the releasing and re-aligning of the body begins, learning the *Natural Walk™* becomes easy. Olympic marathon runners have told me that they expected Rolfing® SI to fix their knee problems and increase their performance, but that changing their stride, so the problems wouldn't return, was an unexpected bonus.

With the structure and the movement patterns of your body, it's a chicken-or-the-egg situation. You need to learn how to move so that your leg tracks straight, so that your knee is not torqued and your leg swings out of the pelvis the way it was designed to.

There are times I have to tell people that their ligaments or cartilage might be damaged. Rolfing® SI can't help that, so I send them on to an orthopedic surgeon. If they have a knee that is not tracking correctly, we can treat the underlying cause(s) once the injury is healed. Fortunately for most clients, the problem has not progressed to needing surgery.

The soft tissue of the body is plastic; releasing it allows it to assume a more relaxed and aligned position. With a little education, the bones can begin to move in their optimal pattern. Inevitably, injuries heal and performance improves once the strain is removed.

An Effective Remedy for Leg Cramps

If you are one of the 6 in 10 adults who have experienced leg cramps, you know how painful they are – and how difficult to prevent. You may have tried the mineral supplements, warm showers, Tylenol, electrolyte drinks, and stretching to no avail.

The Deeper Cause

After ruling out drugs such as birth control pills, diuretics, statins along with high heels, rigid shoes, or orthotics, you need to look at what is causing the muscles to continue to tighten and spasm.

If you are like many of my clients, the reoccurring cramps come from the soft tissue in your lower leg being extremely tense. I was one of those men who prided myself on how big, strong, and firm (tense) my calves were. But calf muscles aren't tight from strength; they're tight from tension. Not walking naturally over years means your calf muscles never really get stretched out. It's as if you were going to the gym and doing bicep curls where you only extend 30%. After a few months your biceps would shorten. From years of the leg not being extended behind you as you walk, the calves never get to fully lengthen.

If you are like every adult client I've seen over the years, you lean back when you walk. This is not only inefficient; it also causes you not to extend your calf out behind you. Learning to lean forward from your ankles as you walk or run will begin to stretch your calves better than stretching. It will also prevent future constriction.

A Solution

Walking correctly will help, but you'll have to release the chronic adhesions deep in your calves. Stretching at this point won't do it. Your calves are too tight to stretch. You first must loosen the deeper calf muscles. This means more than the standard massage. You or a therapist needs to breakdown the fascial (connective tissue) adhesions.

It's true that at first there may be some pain in doing this. But I assure you this pain is small compared to the pain of a leg cramp. I use to punch my legs when I had my cramps for just a little relief. The discomfort of getting chronic tension release actually can feel good because you feel something letting go – unlike my punching.

How to Prevent and Heal Shin Splints

As anyone who has had them will tell you, shin splints are painful and persistent. They are caused when your shin muscle (anterior tibialis) tears away from the bone (tibia), and are the most common running injury, representing up to 60% of all overuse injuries to the lower leg.[16] If the true cause is not treated, you are at risk of developing more serious conditions such as plantar fasciitis (tearing of the connective tissue of the bottom of the foot) and stress fractures (small cracks in the bone).

Traditional treatment includes rest, ice, anti-inflammatory drugs, orthotics, range of motion exercise, a neoprene sleeve, and standard physical therapy. But after three decades of treating runners who tried all these methods, I discovered that symptoms might abate for a while, if you don't stress your leg. Inevitably, as you increase the stress on your leg, the symptoms return or some other problem develops.

I was involved with running studies with Arizona State University and Olympic long distant runners, and we discovered two key points in preventing shin splints from recurring. First, we need to realign the runner's body. If their foot was landing improperly because of torsion in the hip, the hip and thigh need releasing. Second, the client had to change what caused the problem in the first place: their stride.

---

[16] http://shinsplints.wikispaces.com/Classification+and+Prevalence

After Rolfing hundreds of runners, many of them elite athletes, **I never saw one** who had a natural stride. It seems that in this country, after puberty, we start leaning back when we walk or run, causing our stride to go out in front of us. This is unnatural and can be catastrophic to the human body.

You are welcome to download a free book on Natural Running (and walking) at www.align.org. Learning to move your legs and body as intended can alleviate shin splints and other running injuries. Many Olympic runners have told me that what they were taught as running gospel not only didn't help them, it made them worse. The simple premise of leaning into gravity propelled them to set new records without injuries.

Realize that your body will continue to adapt to pain and injury until it can't any longer. By then there is a good chance there are several co-causes to your lingering issue, be it shin splints or back pain. Shifting the load to another body part might feel like it works for a while, but what it's really doing is creating more problems. All my clients who needed hip replacements had a cascade of soft tissue and structural issues for years. They all wished they were more aggressive in treating the primary causes. Please do what you need to now, while you can.

Are Your Legs Keeping You Up?

Many years ago, I had a client whose wife would not sleep in the same bed with him because his legs shook violently while he slept. . The medication he took wasn't working, so, desperate, he called me.

About 10% of the US population has Restless Leg Syndrome (RLS), a condition described as a neurological disorder characterized by an irresistible urge to move the body to stop uncomfortable or odd sensations. Before getting Rolfed 40 years ago, my legs would kick when I slept. I later learned that I had RLS. Studying RLS, I realized I also had many of the co-conditions such as ADHD, body tension, general twitching and fibromyalgia (FMS),. A 2008 study found 64% of participants with FMS also had RLS.[17]

There is no genetic condition or infection that is linked to RLS. A few of us tense people seem to have legs that get restless as we sleep—when you think they would be the most relaxed. But what I realized was that, as they lie in bed, the bodies of people with RLS try to relax more by shaking out the tension.

I've never seen a person with RLS who didn't have exceedingly tight legs. Rock hard tight. At best, we could superficially relax, but we can't release the buildup of chronic tension. Normal stretching or massage is not enough to get the chronic tension released.

Healing RLS

"Some doctors express the view that the incidence of restless leg syndrome is exaggerated by manufacturers of drugs used to treat it."[18] There certainly may be some truth to that; the clients who saw me said their drugs did a poor job treating their symptoms. These people wanted to heal the condition, not just treat the symptoms, though. To do that the entire body needs to release its version of Post Traumatic Stress Disorder (PTSD).

Unfortunately, there is no drug that releases tension; it's something the body must do.

---

[17] A lot of people with fibromyalgia (FMS) have sleep disorders, and restless legs syndrome (RLS) is a common one. In a 2008 study, 64% of participants with FMS also had RLS.

[18] Woloshin, Steven; Schwartz, Lisa M. (2006). "Giving Legs to Restless Legs: A Case Study of How the Media Helps Make People Sick". PLoS Medicine 3 (4): e170.

Realize that RLS is not just a neurological issue, it is also a soft tissue condition. Sure, the nerves play a part, but the stress is stored in the soft tissue. Mindfulness Based Stress Reduction can get the most stressed out clients to heal their ailments, including RLS.[19] Mindfulness teaches the body to turn off the survival response of stress so a relaxed state is the body's default. Acupuncture can also be effective at releasing the body and leg tension. Rolfing® SI healed my client so he could once again share a bed with his wife.

Do You Have a Pain in Your Neck?

There is a 16-25% chance that you had neck pain in the past year, particularly if you're a woman. It's not you though, it's your tension. If you get your neck adjusted but the soft tissue[20] is chronically tight, it will just go back out. A neck that has become tight over the years from stress, poor posture, accidents, or sports has formed scar tissue. The nice loose neck you had as a kid is now a tight post.

The Problem

Virtually all neck pain begins in the soft tissue—the muscles, tendons, ligaments, and fascia. Soft tissue tightens and shortens after an injury, due to postural strain, or just from stress. Then soft tissue literally pulls the bones out of alignment. Eventually, it may even cause the cervical discs to deteriorate. This compression may ultimately impinge (pinch) on a nerve causing numbness or shooting pain down the arm.

Soft tissues pulling on the head often cause headaches. Every client I've seen who was suffering from headaches also had a tight neck. Inevitability, when the neck released, the headaches would disappear

---

[19] http://www.journalsleep.org/ViewAbstract.aspx?pid=28592

[20] http://en.wikipedia.org/wiki/Soft_tissue

Acute and Chronic Causes

Accidents will often cause neck pain. Whiplash injuries from automobile accidents can push the vertebra of the neck backwards causing you to lose the natural curve in your neck. Strains to the upper back or shoulders will often cause the neck muscles to tighten as they adapt to the injury.

On a more long-term basis, poor posture can cause the head to stick forward. Your head weighs a good ten pounds. When the head is out of normal position it places a lot of strain on supporting muscles to do a job they weren't designed to do. These muscles were meant to turn the head, not hold it up against gravity. The posture muscles of the neck and back are very small and deep. When our bodies are in balance, the bigger muscles don't need to work much. They don't need to be stronger—they need to let go.

Some anatomists claim that some of your neck muscles are secondary breathing muscles. Actually, you are only meant to use these neck muscles in survival situations such as running for your life. If you continue to use these muscles to hold up the shoulders (in an attempt to get more air in the upper lobes of the lungs), you end up with shoulders up around your ears and the appearance of having no neck.

The Solution

Because of the many layers of muscles and the seven vertebra of the neck, there is a lot of room for maladaptation and tension. Treating the neck pain means regaining suppleness and mobility. If the tightness is recent, a good massage or a chiropractic adjustment might be all you need. If the tension (but not necessarily the pain) has existed for years, you may need to address the chronic tension to treat the recent pain. My recommendation is to always start with the easiest, cheapest, and quickest treatment, then gradually progress up the treatment scale until you achieve the results you want.

A loose neck will often self-correct. A client of mine told me that one day in kickboxing class, she felt something "tweak in her neck," as she put it. But she stretched and kept moving and it immediately got better because her soft tissue was no longer tight.

Your neck does not have the muscle mass of your legs, but you can develop relatively more connective tissue[21] in the neck from holding your head if it's sticking forward. Pulling it back only creates more tension. That was the problem my kickboxing client had. She had quite a thick, short neck before Rolfing® SI. After Rolfing® SI and releasing the tension in her neck (and shoulders), her neck is actually thinner and a bit longer.

If you're like most people, your neck muscles are doing another unintended job: holding your shoulders up. If your collar bones aren't horizontal, your neck is over-worked and you're probably holding your breath. Clients continually tell me that after their shoulders drop from a few sessions of Rolfing® SI, they realize that they were habitually holding their breath—and holding up their shoulders. Standard exercise does not usually alleviate the pain. In the short run, there may be some improvement because you are moving your neck. But neck pain is not caused by weak muscles; it is caused by tension and misalignment that need to be released.

When I get referrals from doctors and dentists for head-pain problems, the neck is usually the cause of it. Every person I have seen with chronic headaches or TMJ[22] had a tight neck. Getting their necks to release was usually the key to getting rid of their pain. There are many great alternative therapies available, but Rolfing® SI may be what gets your neck to release.

Over several decades of treating clients' neck pain as a Rolfer, I've learned that releasing the chronic tension in the head, neck, and upper back does wonders for healing neck pain. For some clients, much of

---

[21] http://en.wikipedia.org/wiki/Connective_tissue

[22] http://en.wikipedia.org/wiki/Temporomandibular_joint

their neck pain comes from their neck adjusting to an imbalance occurring lower in their body. For instance, if one leg is shorter, your back and neck will adjust so your head is level. Years of this adaptation will create strain. You can loosen the neck, but often the pain will continue if the entire body isn't balanced.

Solutions to Hip Pain

The incidence of total hip replacement (THR) in the U.S. is increasing.[23] To date, 2.5 million people in the U.S. have had THR surgeries.[24] We are getting tighter, more stressed, and more inflamed. To reverse these trends, we first need to change our lifestyles and realize we just don't wake up one morning needing a hip replaced.

Hips don't go bad because the muscles are weak. They go bad because the soft tissue from the back to the knees shortens. Leg-length is shortened, and that adds to the problem. In my 35 years of treating hip pain, often the real cause of the hip pain is the opposite hip tightness. The imbalance of the pelvis ends up affecting the less tight side more.

Chronic tension and misalignment of the soft tissue will continue to pull joints out of place. Chiropractic adjustments are great for the immediate joint misalignment, but for chronic issues, chiropractors and osteopaths will suggest methods that release the soft tissue so the need for regular adjustments decreases.

Yoga is great for stretching and teaching the body to relax under stress. Slowly learning to let go, when your tendency is to tighten, can be transformative. For many that is all that is needed. For the more chronic situation, though, you may need someone to help you release more than the hip muscles. The relative order of therapies that release the

---

[23] Jumped by 205 percent in those aged 45 to 54 from 2000 to 2010; http://www.webmd.com/arthritis/news/20150212

[24] http://paindoctor.com/incidence-hip-pain-demographics-economic-impacts

soft tissue from treating acute to more chronic issues is: mindfulness stress reduction, cranial sacral therapy, acupuncture, massage, and then Rolfing®.

Research and clinical evidence suggest a lot of improvement is gained when you remove foods that cause inflammation. Grains (particularly the gluten grains like wheat), sugar, and food with additives are the most common irritants. Many of my clients report there are numerous supplements that help joints. With chronic tension and misalignment, clients say these supplements don't alleviate the problem. Like drugs, they are treating the symptoms, albeit in a more holistic manner.

The first step is to listen to your body. If you have a reoccurring pain, don't assume it will go away on its own. Sure, it might leave for a while, or shift to somewhere else as you compensate for it. But the pain will not leave unless you treat the cause.

Are You Still Suffering from an Auto Accident?

More than six million Americans have auto accidents every year. Months and even years after an accident, many still have pain from it, usually from soft tissue injuries.

The Problem

Even a low-force accident will strain your soft tissue. Unfortunately, your muscles and fascia are often more like dried out rubber bands than the pliable elastic they should be. When you were younger, your soft tissue was more resilient. It's not age, though. It's all the stress you endure that causes your soft tissue to lose its elasticity, so that when it is forcibly stretched—by the force of a car accident, for example—it doesn't return to its original shape.

The first wave of pain is from the immediate trauma and its inflammation. You might even tear tissue. It hurts. Eventually, this pain subsides, but the second wave of pain occurs after the swelling leaves and the scarring begins. This pain can be in the same areas or in completely different areas that you didn't think were affected. The new injury built upon your old injuries (or just tightness from stress) compounds the intensity. The remedies used for the first wave won't work for the second. Neither will exercise or drugs.

The Solution

You need to release the tightness permanently, not just continue to treat the symptoms. In other words, you need to release the chronic as well as the acute tension. If it's been months since your accident and you are still in pain, some of the old tension from before the accident is playing into the stubbornness of the pain. Any old acute injuries of the past that were never fully released or healed, in addition to any chronic tension, are conspiring with your new injury to produce a condition that won't leave.

Once the chronic tension starts letting go, you start to feel better than you would have imagined possible. Over the years, I've had several clients tell me, "That accident was the best thing that ever happened to me! I was living with the chronic tension, not dealing with it, and now I feel better than before the accident."

A Way Out of TMJ Problems

Temporomandibular joints (TMJ[25]) are the two joints in your lower jaw. If you have pain, clicking, clenching, restricted opening of the mouth, headaches, and ear aches, you know about TMJ dysfunction.

The Problem

The jaw not only opens and closes, it moves sideways. In fact, 38% of neurological input to the brain comes from the face, mouth, and the TMJ region. The soft tissue of the head and mouth affects how it moves. If the jaw moves unevenly, its alignment with the teeth can cause your

---

[25] http://en.wikipedia.org/wiki/Temporomandibular_joint

bite to wear unevenly. Over time, this can wear down the joint as well as your teeth.

In my clinic in Arizona, and in our Mindfulness Stress Reduction[26] classes, we saw many clients for TMJ problems. The majority of these people had above average stress and a reduced ability to effectively deal with their stress. Ten million people suffer from TMJ and 90% are women in their childbearing years. Raising kids is hard work.

The Solution

Soon after I started my Rolfing® SI practice in 1980, I began treating dentists, orthodontists, and oral surgeons. These docs quickly saw the connection between TMJ problems and stress, tightening of soft tissue, and misalignment. Through their referrals and my studies, I began seeing quick success in helping TMJ patients.

Re-aligning the TMJ is not much different than re-aligning a runner's knee. With a knee, the muscles and fascia above and below the knee twist the joint. When the soft tissue balance is restored, the knee tracks straight. The same is true of the jaw. When the surrounding soft tissue is released, the jaw and its joint will re-align. In most cases with a series of Rolfing® SI sessions, if the stress and soft tissue is released and the entire structure is realigned, the pain and associated problems are able to heal. Usually, the joints haven't been destroyed so they tend to fix themselves.

Rolfing® SI doesn't necessarily have to be the therapy used, but TMJ sufferers need to release the tension, restore their alignment, and they must learn a better way to deal with stress. These are all keys to healing TMJ pain.

---

[26] http://stressbeaters.com/

Owen Marcus

Your Hard Stomach Is Making You Sick

Do you have digestive or Genitourinary (urinal or genital) problems? When you gently push on your stomach, does it give or is it firm?

Everything from ulcerative colitis to irritable bowels is linked to chronic stress. Stress is the unfortunate consequence of our 24/7 society. When you're always "on," your body thinks you're in survival mode and acts accordingly: in a crisis, your resources are allocated to the aspects of your body that can save your life, such as your skeletal muscles, while taking from less critical areas such as your digestive system.

Over time the stress and tension accumulate to create tense abs and an internal kink in your GI tract.[27] Your entire abdomen becomes tense, but usually one particular organ takes the hit. For example, the upper abdomen may be so tense and held in that it literally pushes the stomach and esophagus up into your chest causing gastroesophageal reflux[28] or acid reflux, wherein stomach contents back up from the stomach into the esophagus. This also causes the loss of your ability to take a full breath.

No one would intentionally restrict his/her organs, compress his back, or decrease her breath, so why do you do it? You were taught to suck in your gut to look good. Unfortunately, the soft tissue of your gut also became the repository of your stress.

A Solution

I have rarely seen any one come in—not even a child—who doesn't have some tension in his/her abdomen.

---

[27] http://en.wikipedia.org/wiki/Human_gastrointestinal_tract

[28] http://en.wikipedia.org/wiki/Gastroesophageal_reflux_disease

Recently a teenager came to me for neck problems. When I touched her stomach it was like touching her ribcage. There was no give. Her abdomen didn't move as she breathed.

I asked her if she ever had digestive problems. Immediately she began telling me about how she's always in pain. Her symptoms included diarrhea, upset stomach, and menstrual cramps. For years, she saw a series of physicians to diagnosis and treat her problems.

Even though her abdomen felt like a rock, we were able to get it to release a little. A week later she returned to tell me she had no abdominal symptoms. The physical release of her tension, coupled with her practicing letting her stomach relax began to give her organs more space.

Therapies

The key to turning around visceral problems that result from soft tissue tensions is getting the tissue to release. If the problem is recent, subtler therapies like acupuncture and visceral manipulation may be all you need. But if the problem has existed for years and the abdomen is hard, a more direct therapy like abdominal massage or Rolfing® SI will yield better results.

I have seen amazing results with both acupuncture and the gentle visceral manipulation taught by the French physician Jean-Pierre Barral. Many years ago I took one of the first classes Dr. Barral taught here in the U.S. When the abdomen is relaxed, the slightest pressure from a skilled hand can release the tension around an organ allowing it to resume normal functioning.

There are massage therapists who teach abdominal massage. Many of these massage techniques come from oriental massage practices such as Thai massage.[29]

---

[29] http://en.wikipedia.org/wiki/Thai_massage

A Certified Rolfer's™ goal is not only to remove the direct and indirect strain, but to educate the client on how to relax in order to guarantee that the problem not only leaves, but never returns. The amazing thing about soft tissue is that it will release. The trick is getting it to release so the body reorganizes to prevent the same problem—or a new one. When that happens there can be many positive unintended consequences, such as the return of a regular menstrual cycle in women who had previously blamed running for the lack of one.

Rolfing® SI and Irritable Bowel Syndrome (IBS)

Over the years, many of the clients who saw me for musculo-skeletal problems also reported having Irritable Bowel Syndrome[30] (IBS). In every case, these clients' abdomens were tenser than the norm. Up to 50% of gastroenterology referrals are related to this syndrome.[31]

As a Certified Rolfer™, I view the body as parts that are all interconnected. Systemic tension and misalignment throughout the body can cause gut tension. The converse is also true; your gut tension will produce strain in your musculoskeletal system, as my study of visceral manipulation (releasing tension specific to organs) showed me. It's as if each organ is a balloon attached to other balloons that are attached to the inner abdominal wall. The tension of the body can affect the structure and positioning of one of these organ balloons, pulling them out of position, which will affect the organ's function.

What Does Stress Do?

Beyond structural stress, any emotional or physiological stress compounds the problem. Emotional stress builds up in your soft tissue, and your guts are all soft tissue. The soft tissue of your abdomen can become an emotional reservoir for chronic stress. If you hold on to your

---

[30] http://en.wikipedia.org/wiki/Irritable_bowel_syndrome

[31] Jenifer K Lehrer, MD, eMedicine Specialties, Gastroenterology, Colon

feelings, you hold your guts tensely. Since the colon is partly controlled by the autonomic nervous system[32] (the survival, or fight-or-flight[33] nervous system) we are inescapably inclined to store chronic stress in our gut. This constant irritation creates inflammation, which produces an immune response, which many researchers tie to IBS.

Trauma, both physical and emotional, can set up IBS. The physical trauma of an injury or surgery can create structural strain that affects the colon. Emotional trauma can produce post traumatic stress disorder[34] (PTSD) that continually produces tension on the brain-gut axis.

What Is The Solution?

If structural or emotional stress is part of the cause of your IBS, you need to release that stress to achieve sustainable results. Creating a relaxed stomach is part of this. I know what you're thinking: we're supposed to have a tight stomach, right? What about rock-hard abs? Six-packs? But a tight, hard gut is not healthy. Babies and animals don't have tense stomachs; adults do because of stress and aesthetics. In spite of our cultural training, we aren't meant to have hard stomachs. Six-pack abs is a set-up for visceral and back problems. Abdominal tension not only compresses you by shortening your waist, it compresses your organs. It is as if you have someone sitting on your stomach. Whatever therapy you choose, you will also need to consciously practice relaxing your stomach. As easy as that might seem, it will take some practice relaxing and some intent to let go of your cultural belief that a hard, tight, and muscular abdomen is desirable.

Often the biggest hurdle to helping my clients getting well is getting them to relax their stomachs so they breathe deeper, giving their organs more room and getting their deep back muscles to relax. I also tell

---

[32] http://en.wikipedia.org/wiki/Autonomic_nervous_system

[33] http://en.wikipedia.org/wiki/Fight-or-flight_response

[34] http://en.wikipedia.org/wiki/Posttraumatic_stress_disorder

them not to do sits-ups or crunches until they master breathing with their bellies.

When I had my clinic in Scottsdale, AZ, where we ran our Mindfulness Stress Reduction courses, a lot of students came to us with IBS. By learning to relax—particularly, by relaxing their stomachs—their conditions would improve or disappear.

Physical manipulation, such as Rolfing® SI, is the short cut to getting your stomach to relax and stay relaxed, thereby allowing your bowel to heal. No part of your body can fully heal if it is under stress. Its resources are diverted to what it experiences as survival, rather than to healing.

Take a deep breath, breathe into your abdomen, relax your stomach ... you are now on the road to healing your IBS.

A Rolfer's™ Perspective on Sciatica

Nearly everyone I know has experienced a form of low back pain at least one time in their lives. This pain is most often centered around the sacrum, hip bones, and sacroiliac joints, with pain radiating downward through the backside and into the thighs and calves. This radiating pain is often suddenly sharp and can be so severe it puts us down and out for days waiting for recovery.

The Problem

The cause of such horrible pain arises from pressure or compression on the sciatic nerve[35], the longest nerve in the body that runs from the lower spine through the pelvis and gluteal muscles, angling down to the back sides of the lower legs. With this intermittent or chronic pain,

---

[35] http://en.wikipedia.org/wiki/Sciatic_nerve

there may also be numbness and tingling in the legs, feet, and toes as nerve transmission becomes reduced.

Many causes of compression on the sciatic nerve have been identified. One cause could originate from muscle tension, especially the piriformis muscle[36] that originates on the side of the sacrum, crosses over the sciatic nerve as it angles across the pelvis, and attaches on the hip bone. Heavy lifting, twisting, perhaps long hours driving or prolonged positions in front of your computers without frequent stretching, or general overwork of the pelvic and hip muscles can generate a spasm of the piriformis and compression on the sciatic nerve.

As the sciatic nerve exits from the spinal column, any damage, wear and tear, tumors, protrusions, or bulges to the discs—our shock absorbers—can reduce spinal flexibility, all of which can lead to an irritation or pressure on the sciatic nerve root. Spinal misalignment can become an accessory to sciatic pain.

When these familiar pains remain unaddressed, the body often develops adaptive behaviors and positions to compensate for the pain and reduction of flexibility. Over time, this can lead to permanent damage to the discs, the vertebrae, and the affected nerves. Some methods of treatment have been administering pain killing and anti-inflammatory drugs. However, these may also have serious side effects with long-term usage. The use of heat and cold therapies may be suggested along with stretching and strengthening exercises to release spasms and ease pain symptoms. Another therapy has been the use of anti-inflammatory steroid injections to the site, again with the potential of side effects. In serious cases where diagnosis and testing has revealed bone or disc damage, surgery may be the recommended solution.

---

[36] http://en.wikipedia.org/wiki/Piriformis_muscle

Owen Marcus

The Solution

Sciatica[37] is a common problem. Studies estimate that 13% to 40% of adults suffer from it, and 1% to 5% suffer annual recurrences. For more than 30 years now, sciatic pain has been a common reason why clients come to me for Rolfing® SI.

Over the years, I've learned some things about sciatic pain: whether the pain is caused by low back strain, a herniated disc, or hip muscle strain (e.g., piriformis muscle), inevitably the true source is soft tissue strain. The body's muscles and connective tissue (fascia, tendons, and ligaments) contract, pull on the skeleton, yank it out of alignment, and cause pain. This strain compresses the discs of the back, which is the major cause of sciatica. The strain can also force the muscles of the hip to contract (the sciatic nerve travels through those muscles) creating "pseudo-sciatica."

Think of your soft tissue as leather; if it shrinks (tightens up due to injury, stress, or pain), your entire body shortens. The low back is the most vulnerable to shortening because of the large muscles and connective tissue of the deep abdomen and the back muscles.

"No matter what I do for my 'core,' I can't seem to strengthen my lower back or flatten my low abdomen," one of my clients told me. Even when she wasn't having sciatic pain, her low back often just felt tired. No amount of stretching helped, because it wasn't just her muscles that had shortened up; all of her fascia was also too tight. After seeing me for Rolfing® SI, she told me: "It's like my low back muscles woke up." She hasn't had any pain, and she can finally exercise some of those core muscles she had only heard about before. Her stomach is flatter and her back is stronger.

With this shortening, your organs and back are susceptible to impairment, as are the nerves that run out of the spine. Your discs are like the

---

[37] http://en.wikipedia.org/wiki/Sciatica

jelly in jelly donuts, filling in the space between the vertebrae of the back, allowing the back to bend. After years of strain, these discs flatten into pancakes and the low back shortens. (This is where we lose most of our height.) Then the compressed discs can bulge, pushing against a nerve. In the hip, the deep hip muscles can contract around the nerve.

The compounded strain over the years distorts your entire structure, forcing your bones to try to compensate, essentially mal-forming your skeleton. If your body's entire leather suit shrinks, your skeleton does the best job it can to adjust to the decreasing space. But your nerves are very sensitive to irritation from this chronic imbalance. We can fix one part of this puzzle, but if the systemic strain remains, you will have recurring pain.

Fortunately, the whole process is reversible. Think of it like straightening out a twisted hose. You can't just straighten out one section; you need to unwind the torque from the entire hose so it will lie flat. To stretch out your soft tissue, so your skeleton can go back to its natural state, you have to "unwind" all the soft tissue, releasing the chronic stress and allowing your body to regain its natural state.

All your soft tissue needs releasing—not only where the pain is located, but throughout your entire body—for significant lasting change. There are many ways to get a release; Rolfing® SI is just one of them.

What Is Behind Your Shoulder Pain

In 2003, 13.7 million Americans saw physicians for shoulder problems. So chances are, even if you don't have a shoulder problem, you know someone who does.

Most common shoulder conditions are sore rotator cuffs (tendonitis or bursitis) and frozen shoulders (caused by adhesions that restrict motion). Both are soft tissue issues—problems in the muscle and fascia (the connective tissue holding the muscles together).

At my clinic in Scottsdale, I got a lot of referrals from a hand surgeon. This particular surgeon got the patients that no other doctor could help.

He was not a big fan of shoulder surgery, though; he believed that most of these problems could be solved through treating the soft tissue—and he was right. In every case I saw, the patient's pain was caused by an improperly positioned arm. When their arm was de-rotated, their pain disappeared.

When you stand in front of a mirror, which way does your elbow point? When you bend your arm, the lower arm should raise up in front of your stomach. Just as your knees are meant to point forward, your elbows are meant to point out to the side. If your elbow points behind you, your arm is misaligned.

The Problem

The shoulder joint[38] is amazing. Soft tissue is all that holds together the actual joint, which is the most mobile joint in the body, and the shoulder girdle (shoulder blade and collar bone). This huge range of motion allows you to tuck your shirt in, throw a baseball, and climb a tree. But it also makes the shoulder joint vulnerable to injury.

Over years of using the arm in ways it wasn't designed, or as the result of previous injuries, scar tissue builds up. Each little strain is a microtrauma that produces a little more scar tissue. The scar tissue helps stabilize and protect the joint, but it also pulls the arm and shoulder out of alignment, producing more strain. Often this pattern shortens the back of the joint and weakens the front, setting the joint up for a rotator cuff[39] injury. Or the entire joint might tighten up, producing a frozen shoulder.

---

[38] http://en.wikipedia.org/wiki/Shoulder

[39] http://en.wikipedia.org/wiki/Rotator_cuff

The Solution

Without putting the arm into proper alignment, the arm and shoulder will always be vulnerable to injury no matter what treatment you use. To fix the current problem and prevent future injuries, the entire arm and shoulder need to be structurally re-organized.

This sounds more complicated than it usually is. First, the soft tissue restrictions need to be released from the neck to the mid-back and out to the shoulder joint. (The infraspinatus, a muscle in the back of the shoulder blade, is usually twisting the arm.) Often, restriction in the arm needs releasing, but it needs to be done with an eye to re-establishing proper alignment, not just relaxing all the muscles.

Once all the soft tissue regains its resiliency and everything is back in position, the shoulder pain disappears. Of course, you'll need to learn how to use your arm correctly, so as not to recreate the strain: whenever possible, bend your arm with the elbow out to the side. For example, don't do bicep curls with your elbow pointing back; do them with your elbow on your knee, pointing out to the side.

I've treated baseball pitchers who were looking at giving up their career because of shoulder injuries. In every case—and often after only one session—they were pitching faster and more accurately than ever as a result of Rolfing® SI. The body has an amazing ability to heal itself when the strain is removed and its natural order is returned.

If you're wondering whether this is all related to tennis elbow and carpal tunnel injuries, the answer is yes. The rotation that causes chronic shoulder problems causes those, too.

Yoga for Shoulder and Orthopedic Problems

If you ever had a shoulder injury you know how frustrating it can be, let alone how painful. You get to the point where you can barely use the arm. That is not good.

Over the years, I have had over a hundred clients with frozen shoulders or rotator cuff injuries[40], often referred by orthopedic surgeons. For Certified Rolfers™ it is one of the easiest problems to fix. Until this article in the New York Times[41], I've never heard anyone else mention the secret to healing shoulder injuries.

The supraspinatus muscle[42] on the back of the shoulder blade gets tight and short as it turns into scar tissue as a result of the arm being constantly rotated out. When your elbow points behind you and not out to the side, this little muscle is to blame.

Loren Fishman, a physiatrist (physical and rehabilitative medicine specialist) affiliated with New York-Presbyterian/Columbia Hospital, built upon his yoga training to create a simple stretch to release this muscle. Read his New York Times article, "Ancient Moves for Orthopedic Problems" to learn how you can heal your bad shoulder.

Expanding Our Medical View

As a Certified Rolfer™, clients often see me after, having seen a series of physicians, they are still in pain. I know these docs want to help their patients. The problem is not doctors, it is our medical system. David Katz, M.D., Director of Yale University's Prevention Research Center claims, in this post[43], that the limits of medicine's understanding can limit the care a patient receives.

---

[40] http://en.wikipedia.org/wiki/Rotator_cuff

[41] http://www.nytimes.com/2011/08/02/health/02brody.html?_r=2

[42] http://en.wikipedia.org/wiki/Supraspinatus_muscle

[43] http://www.huffingtonpost.com/david-katz-md/rolling-our-eyes-at-our-p_b_685998.html

As reported by *The New York Times*[44], a fascinating study published in the *Journal of Neuropathology and Experimental Neurology*[45] suggests that even Lou Gehrig may not have had Lou Gehrig's disease.[46] Rather, it's possible that Gehrig had progressive, neurological deterioration mimicking amyotrophic lateral sclerosis (ALS) due to head trauma[47] (among other things, he was hit in the head by a fastball).

The first physician I treated was a physiatrist (a physical medicine specialist—i.e. if a physical therapist was an MD, he would be a physiatrist). One of the first things he told me was that there was no medical test to measure soft tissue injuries or the associated pain. He said this as a leader in the field of thermography (thermal imaging), which is possibly the only known method to evaluate soft tissue.

Medicine and its tests don't measure soft tissue problems, like pain or stress—the key areas Certified Rolfers™ treat. I encourage you to not limit yourself by what medical tests say or don't say. Listen to your body, seek second options beyond physicians.

Dr. Andrew Weil on Rolfing®SI

There is a blog post[48] by Andrew Weil, MD[49] on the four reasons to try Rolfing® SI. His four are pain and stress, improving your posture, releasing repressed emotions, and diminishing habitual muscle tension, and

---

[44] http://www.nytimes.com/2010/08/18/sports/18gehrig.html?_r=1&emc=na

[45] http://journals.lww.com/jneuropath/Documents/tdp-43%2520proteinopathy%2520and%2520motor%2520neuron%2520disease%2520in%2520chronic%2520traumatic%2520encephalopathy.pdf

[46] http://en.wikipedia.org/wiki/Amyotrophic_lateral_sclerosis

[47] http://en.wikipedia.org/wiki/Head_injury

[48] http://www.drweil.com/drw/u/TIP02924/Four-Reasons-to-Try-Rolfing.html

[49] http://www.drweil.com/

they match my three reasons of stress, structural issues, and soft tissue issues.

Dr. Weil is a great spokesperson for holistic health. Many years ago, my business partner and I brought Dr. Weil in to help us with the creation of our *Scottsdale Institute for Health and Medicine*. I first met him when he was a keynote speaker back in the early 80's for a Rolf® SI Institute conference. He continues to impress me with his ability to articulate the benefits of holistic health. His book[50] on the healthcare crisis is right-on. As he says, "We don't have a healthcare system here in the US; we have a disease management system—and it doesn't work."

How to Turn Around Fibromyalgia Syndrome (FMS)

Oftentimes, patients receive feedback from health care providers that what they are experiencing is "all in their heads" or that they are "hypochondriacs." This happens when traditional medicine is unable to identify specific clues and explanations for the patient's discomfort. Fibromyalgia has often been classified by doctors as "all in your head." I have however, found fibromyalgia to be curable with the correct combination of therapies." In some cases, they have experienced a series of diagnoses and treatments that have just not proven beneficial for them over time.

Fibromyalgia Is Not a Disease

I have found fibromyalgia to be curable with the correct combination of therapies. As I mentioned in the post on www.stressedout.org, the medical profession fails to recognize fibromyalgia as a real problem because they believe they have a drug for it. As you read up on this drug,

---

[50] http://www.amazon.com/Why-Our-Health-Matters-Transform/dp/1594630666

you will find that the drug company is not promising a cure, just a mitigation of symptoms.

Fibromyalgia Syndrome presents as chronic muscular and joint pain that causes widespread body achiness with tenderness at various points on the body. This achiness tends to move around and therefore becomes hard to pinpoint, sometimes reflecting a burning sensation and/or a tingling sensation. Sufferers may also complain of loss of sleep, low energy, stiffness following rest times, or a lack of feeling rested after a night's sleep. It is often greatly debilitating. Mostly, FMS causes a general all-over body ache and constant pain and discomfort—a condition that affects one's overall well-being and ability to function fully.

FMS symptoms often overlap with other disorders such as Chronic Fatigue Syndrome, Irritable Bowel Syndrome, Hypothyroidism (low thyroid function), Sleep Disorder, and/or TMJ dysfunction (if pain first shows up in the jaw area). This is why FMS is so hard to pin down for the medical community.

The most important therapeutic direction focuses on the management of FMS and on learning all one can about what is being experienced—paying attention to body signals, timing, and relative intensity at various times throughout the day.

Releasing Stress Heals Fibromyalgia

Do you have ongoing, non-specific pain? Is this pain worse when you are tired or stressed? If you answered yes, you may be suffering from fibromyalgia. I wrote a post on fibromyalgia for my StressedOut.org blog explaining fibromyalgia and its relationship to stress. This post is the most read post on that blog. Fibromyalgia is a hot topic.

For years, I have told my clients that as a culture we live on the fibromyalgia continuum. Virtually everyone is at least developing some of the symptoms. The subclinical symptoms may only show up sporadically when we have pushed ourselves for several days.

Chronic sufferers of fibromyalgia just didn't suddenly catch the condition. Fibromyalgia comes from our bodies being progressively run down. Years of stress, working hard, not getting enough rest, and poor nutrition are some of the factors that can lead to the physiological exhaustion which develops into fibromyalgia.

Exhausted and Hyper

What is interesting from a clinical prospective is that all of the diagnosed fibromyalgia sufferers I have seen in my practice are wired and exhausted. Most often, their soft tissue is lacking life or as an oriental medical doc would say, has low chi. Their deeper soft tissue is tense and fibrous. Many of these clients are committed to getting well and have seen many other good practitioners without getting well. These docs and healthcare providers, along with the clients, can't understand why they are still sick.

Just as with depression and chronic fatigue, which are closely related to fibromyalgia, fibromyalgia clients need to release the deep chronic tension to get well. That deeper layer of soft tissue needs to come back to life. It is as if that layer is blocking the chi and blood circulation from reaching vital organs and the more superficial levels.

From my experience, if a person truly wants to get well from fibromyalgia and is willing to step outside the normal treatment box, he/she will get well. The road back to wellness will take a while. It will require commitment and a willingness to feel and express old emotions. There will be times when the person will feel worse (this is called a "healing crisis"), and will be more exhausted, depressed, and/or have more short-term pain. By hanging in there, *you will get well*.

Chronic Fatigue – Other Options

If you are one of the 800,000+ adults in the USA with Chronic Fatigue Syndrome[51] (CFS), you know how miserable you feel and how many will tell you to learn to live with it—or worse, that you are just lazy. CFS is one of those chronic illnesses Andrew Weil, MD, speaks about when he says medicine is useless in healing and holistic health offers many possibilities.

Causes

One cause that gets little attention because it is not an external cause—and in my experience it is the most frequent culprit—is chronic stress and/or Post Traumatic Stress Disorder (PTSD). Over years of dealing with constant stress, experienced as a survival response, your body gets worn down. I don't care how strong you are; at some point continual exposure to stress will exhaust your body.

We are not designed to always have our resources oriented towards survival. Something will give. For some, it is depression, for others it is fibromyalgia, and for many it is CFS. It is no surprise that medical research has linked the three. I have seen patients who were unfortunate enough to suffer from all three.

There can be biological co-causes such as toxicity and nutritional deficiencies. Twenty years ago I had a client who was referred to me after several years of medical and holistic treatment. She was tense, exhausted, and so frustrated that she flushed all her psychotropic drugs[52] down the toilet. We discovered that part of her problem was that her father had dumped his old dry-cleaning fluid in the same backyard that she played in. With the Rolfing® SI and a detox program, she was feeling better within a month. In six months, she felt better than she had ever felt.

---

[51] http://en.wikipedia.org/wiki/Chronic_fatigue_syndrome

[52] http://en.wikipedia.org/wiki/Psychoactive_drug

Solutions

First, release the chronic stress. Good bodywork such as Rolfing® SI, skilled massage, or possibly acupuncture will allow the old, deep tension to release. Slow-yoga, where you are learning to relax, can help as well as a Mindfulness Stress Reduction Program.[53] Second, find a qualified holistic practitioner who can guide you through detoxing your body and rebuilding it. She may be a nutritionist, herbalist, naturopath, or acupuncturist. It matters less what type of healing she practices than the fact that you feel comfortable with her, and that she has experience successfully treating CFS.

So often my CFS patients tell me they are exhausted, but they can't sleep. They can't sleep because their nervous system is wired. Sleeping pills or antidepressants don't release that tension. Releasing the physical tension in the body will relax the nervous system. Once the body relaxes and escapes the constant state of "fight or flight," (due to what is ultimately caused by PTSD), the body shifts its resources from survival to healing.

Without PTSD or stress, your body will slowly heal and regenerate. You may feel more tired as you relax and as your body recovers from years of stress. Allow yourself the rest you need. I've seen clients sleep twelve plus hours a night until they started to catch up. Your body has an amazing ability to heal when it feels safe, healthy, rested, and nourished.

The Power of Rolfing® SI

Over the 30 years I have treated people, I have received many referrals from others who normally get great results, but who were not getting them for these types of clients. We all learned that without releasing these deep layers, it is as if other work, such as homeopathy and clinical nutrition, can't get into the tissue. Once the stress, exhaustion, and ten-

---

[53] http://en.wikipedia.org/wiki/Mindfulness-based_stress_reduction

sion releases, previously ineffective therapies begin to work better than they had. These clients often prove to be some of the most successful cases for other practitioners. Rolfing® SI can free the body to allow other therapies to support deep healing and rejuvenation.

A Rolfer's™ trained touch knows how to stimulate the autonomic nervous system in a gentle way so there is enough arousal to activate the system, yet not too much to cause anything close to a fight or flight response. Once activated, that tense or charged area is able to let go. Over the course of one session this may happen hundreds of times, discharging the entire body and training the body how to do this on its own. A body that once responded to even pleasant stimuli with a stress response can learn to release a stress response as it occurs.

A Different Approach to Back Pain

It's inevitable. Like death and taxes. Back pain.

Second to colds, the most likely reason you'll visit a healthcare provider will be back pain. At least 50% of Americans report back pain each year.

Are you in pain right now? Is your movement limited? Are you reducing your activities because of the pain or the fear of the pain? Let's look at the reasons:

A lot of back pain comes from overexertion. If that's you, you're lucky. Your pain will go away once your body recovers from being pushed. And there's a good chance it won't return—unless you overdo it again. In time, you'll be fine.

For pain due to overexertion, traditional remedies work well. Cold compresses can reduce swelling. Warm, moist heat helps muscles that feel tight, relax. Alternating the two can be beneficial. And of course, massage and gentle stretching relax the tightness, and the movement prevents further stiffness. Rest always supports the body in healing. Topical ointments will give you warmth and local pain relief.

Chronic Back Pain

Chronic back pain is a different animal. Pain often occurs without physical exertion; it just shows up. As the frequency and intensity of episodes increase, each incident leaves a tension residue that sets up the next attack of pain. Pain pills and muscle relaxers may help, but many people don't like their side effects. One thing is clear: just treating the symptom is not enough—particularly when the problem is likely to return.

What They Don't Tell You About Back Pain

When half of working Americans admit to having back pain every year, you know there is a problem that's not being solved.[54] The standard belief is that back pain comes from tight back muscles or a nerve being pitched. Therefore, solving the problem simply requires relaxing those back muscles, or surgery on the nerve impingement.

One day you're fine, the next day you roll out of bed unable to stand up. In dire pain, incapable of walking, you crawl to the phone to get someone to drive you to your doc for drugs to relax the muscles and relieve the pain. And they work. For a while the pain subsides... if you're lucky. The first time it happens, you convince yourself that the back pain was a fluke. You have a vague memory of a twinge when you sneezed, and the next day you woke in excruciating pain, but lightning can't strike twice, right?

But realistically, your first bout of back pain was an omen for more. If you're smart, you get proactive. Maybe you see doctors or other medical professionals. Some tell you that you have a disc that is not right. Others tell you that your back muscles are tight. Someone might tell you that you're just too stressed. You might try all their solutions: surgery, stretching, and stress reduction... but your pain returns.

---

[54] Vallfors B. Acute, Subacute and Chronic Low Back Pain: Clinical Symptoms, Absenteeism and Working Environment. Scan J Rehab Med Suppl 1985; 11: 1-98.

Many repeated acute back pain incidences are really a reflection of chronic tension, structural misalignment, and maladaptive movement patterns. In over 30 years of seeing clients with back pain, even the acute cases could be traced back to a chronic situation. My clients learn that where it hurts is not the root of their pain. At best, treating the pain area relieves the pain temporarily. If these clients haven't figured it out yet, they quickly realize that other areas—such as their tight stomach and pelvis—cause their back muscles to tighten in reaction to these stronger areas tightening.

Many years ago, a surgeon was referred to me by his associate. He came to me for his chronic back pain. After quoting studies his colleagues did on the effectiveness of back surgery, he admitted, "I am looking at things I would have never considered before." I showed him how it was only natural that his back muscles were in constant spasm because his abdominal muscles, pelvis muscles and even the fascia (connective tissue) of his legs were shortening his back. Showing how his ribcage was inside his pelvis (when optimally it should be three-fingers width above it) he got it. When all these chronically tense areas released and straightened out, his back was better than it had been for decades.

Misconceptions on Back Pain

We all know to use our legs when lifting heavy objects, but that's really all we're taught about how to keep our backs healthy. But when you acknowledge that back problems don't originate in the back, you learn that there are many ways to prevent back pain. In more than 30 years of Rolfing® SI®, I've never seen anyone with acute or chronic back issues who wasn't tense in their abdomen, pelvis and legs. When these structures release, often the back releases.

The first thing I tell my clients is, forget all that you learned about good posture—because it's wrong. Yes, you want to start straight, but not at the cost of creating tension. The old adage, "Shoulders back, stomach in, chest out, and feet straight" is not a natural stance even for the loosest and best-aligned individual. That stance will have the back muscles being posture muscles, a job they aren't designed to do.

To maintain a relaxed abdomen, STOP holding your gut in. Holding your stomach in restricts your breath. It also will restrict rib movement, a setup for upper back problems. Breathe. Let your stomach relax – which is the best way to release stress. Give your organs and back some room.

Stop fighting gravity. You will never win. Have someone take a profile picture of you. See how, in spite of feeling aligned, you are leaning back. That leaning back compresses the lower back and makes your soft tissue system do jobs it's not meant to do. That constant stress causes serial micro-traumas to your body, creating more constricting connective tissue.

The best way to shift the backward tilt is to learn how to walk naturally. Lean into gravity, allowing what was once shortening muscles to lengthen. You can download a free book on Natural Running and Walking at: www.align.org.

Minimize the effect of long sitting by sitting on your sits bone, thereby allowing your back to be vertical. The slouching most people do compresses the back and sticks your head out. Having your furniture fit you, rather than you fit it, will, over time make a huge difference. Invest in a good ergonomic chair that supports this good posture.

Another misconception is that to have a strong back, you need strong abdominal muscles. Most people will feel an initial improvement from doing sit ups, because you are moving and learning a new way to compensate. Yet over time, you are using another set of muscles to do a job they aren't meant to do. Moreover, you are further compressing the space between your ribcage and pelvis. Your discs go from being jelly donuts to pancakes.

Relax. Relax, relax, relax. Let your body do what comes naturally. Stop fighting gravity, and stop fighting your own body.

Prevention and Treatment

The best way to treat chronic back pain is to prevent it. Learn to lift using your legs. Sit on your sits bones. Stop slouching! It will all reduce back strain. Use ergonomic furniture that adjusts to your unique body, instead of forcing your body to adapt to the furniture. Moving helps, too—get up and walk around, take breaks.

And the most critical behavior—the one we never think about—is breathing. I know, you are breathing. The question is: How well are you breathing?

When I taught Mindfulness Stress Reduction courses in Scottsdale, AZ, the principal reason people came to us was back pain. At the time, we were the largest company offering these courses in the country. Most of our students for the 8-week course were referrals from hospital networks or corporate clients.

We taught the students to breathe. As easy as it might sound, the first few weeks were tough. Very simple relaxation exercises would actually create stress. The students' old habits prevented them from relaxing and breathing fully. Once they realized their tension, they saw how much they were limiting their breath—even when they believed they were relaxed. With daily homework and coming to the weekly class, their awareness and the quality of their breathing increased as their stress and pain declined.

What does this mean for you? If these very tense people can dramatically change their stress and pain in 8-weeks, so can you. The first step is to become aware of how you hold your body and your breath. If you are holding one, you are holding the other. As your breath becomes fuller, slower, and more relaxed, you begin to train your body not to hold stress, but to release it.

In keeping with letting go, I suggest to my clients that they do not do "back strengthening" exercises. I have not seen a back that was muscularly weak; I see many that are structurally weak. Our bigger back muscles are not meant to be posture muscles, they are designed to move us, not hold us. The constant holding makes them tighter. Rather than getting stronger from sit-ups or back extensions, practice breathing and stretching.

There's an 80% Chance You Will See Your Doc About Back Pain During Your Life.

As a Certified Rolfer™, I tend to treat people after they have tried everything else. This is not because other treatments are ineffective—it's because the tension that is causing the persistent problem is old. After many years of repeated back problems, the entire body gets tighter and more distorted. The original problem might have stemmed from a childhood injury. Over the years, the body experiences more stress and injury, and develops patterns of compensation that all add to increased tension. At some point, the body exhausts its ability to counteract the original strain pattern. Now you are worse off—you have the original tension plus years of coping with it.

The Often-Overlooked Source of Back Pain

We all know we get shorter as we age. But it's not our bones shortening—it's the soft tissue shortening and screwing down. Here is a quick test to evaluate what your low back is up against:

- Stand up, and place your fingers on your pelvis.

- Push in a little with your thumb until you feel that lowest twelfth rib.

- Optimally, you should have the space of three finger widths between your pelvis and your lowest rib.

Rarely do I find that much space. Two finger widths is great, one is adequate. When you are at no space or your ribs are actually inside your pelvis, you have a problem.

This is where we lose most of our height. Remember, our discs are like the jelly in jelly donuts, filling the space between the vertebrae, allowing the spine to move. They become pancakes from this compression.

When the discs compress and the tissue around them tightens, they dehydrate from lack of circulation and movement. This sets up bulging or ruptured discs that may require surgery. This chronic tension and shortness just makes you more vulnerable to back injury and pain.

Strengthening your back will often give you short-term gains; you'll have increased movement, and you may develop a new pattern of compensation. Over time, the soft tissue just gets tighter. We need to go in the other direction. We need to release and lengthen the tissue. Unfortunately at this point, stretching does not work for most people. Stretching these muscles is like stretching a steel cable. We need to make the soft tissue soft again.

What Is Possible

If the body created soft tissue strain, it can usually un-create it. When the correct amount of pressure is applied to the right area, the tissue begins to release. Over time, hydration, subtleness, and movement returns. The body begins to unwind as it lengthens out. The space in between the pelvis and the ribs reappears.

Once the body attains a level of order and relaxation, the change becomes sustainable. Our bodies prefer pleasure to pain. When we are so used to pain, it can take a while for our bodies to trust that our backs can be as they were when we were younger.

Part of returning this vibrancy to our tissue comes from changing simple behaviors. The first is learning not to protect your back. The natural behavior of holding to avoid or reduce your back pain over time only makes your back tighter. I have seen people whose pain is long gone, whose backs are loose, but who still protect out of habit. Noticing how subtly we hold is huge. A little bit of constant holding over a long period of time adds up to a significant amount of holding. A lot of subtle letting go adds up also.

Rolfing® SI is certainly not the only means to releasing chronic tension, but it may be the quickest. Teaching the entire body to deeply and consistently relax has many benefits. Learning to breathe and dealing with stress can significantly improve chronic pain.

An Alternative Perspective on Scoliosis

We all know someone who has scoliosis.[55] Chances are it is a girl or a woman who developed it around puberty. This idiopathic (unknown cause) form is more common than the congenital form which starts earlier in life.

Treating the twist usually involves one of three approaches. The least invasive is exercise or physical therapy, the next requires braces, and the last resort is surgery, which entails insertion of a Harrington rod[56] in the spine.

To understand the consequences of these approaches, we must understand what is pulling the vertebrae out of alignment. The skeleton sits in a web of soft tissue and the 650 plus muscles are just a part of this web.

A New Twist on Treatment

Rather than attempting to pull the spine back in place by tightening other soft tissue through exercise and bracing or inserting a steel rod, it is best to determine what is pulling the vertebrae out of place and release those tightened soft tissues.

Particularly when the young adolescent is first developing scoliosis, the body is amenable to letting go of its tension. Sheets of fascia hold everything together and travel beyond individual muscles. This means that tension or imbalance in the legs will affect the back, first by causing an uneven base for the spine, then also from the uneven pull.

---

[55] http://en.wikipedia.org/wiki/Scoliosis

[56] http://en.wikipedia.org/wiki/Harrington_implant

Not only is releasing the soft tissue strain the least invasive approach, it can be the most sustainable. If the strain is gone, then the chance of the curve returning is gone, just like patching a crack in a wall by first leveling the foundation allows the patch to last.

Twenty years ago, a physician referred a middle-aged woman who had developed scoliosis as a teenager to me for Rolfing® SI. She came back for her fourth session telling me that an x-ray her doc had taken showed an improvement. After her tenth session, I took a set of Polaroid pictures to compare to her "before" photos. She was standing straight. Yes, if you looked closely you could see a small curve, but with clothes on she looked straighter than most.

Upon viewing her before and after photos, she found it hard to believe she was really straight after all those years of suffering with scoliosis. Working with the soft tissue causes for skeletal misalignment is often one of the best solutions for the correction of this condition. The bodies can be more plastic than our minds in their ability to adapt to higher states of order.

Owen Marcus

Expanding Our Concepts

Discover What Is Possible from a
New Perspective in Alternative Therapies

Rolfing® SI is based on common sense assumptions backed up with years of clinical evidence and a growing body of research.[57] A Certified Rolfer's™ approach to a body is unique. When we first started speaking about these principles many thought it was strange.

For example, 40 years ago we were speaking about the importance of our core muscles. Now every gym talks about it. Unfortunately, as with other principles, something was lost in the translation to the general public. Core strength is not about tightening your deep muscles. It's often first about releasing them, which allows you to fully access them so they are able to perform as intended. Then it's about learning to balance the use of your core muscles with your more extrinsic (outer) muscles.

Pilates is best known for teaching its clients to use their core muscles. When a person is able to access and utilize their deeper core muscles and the structures around them because they are free—and because they are aligned—the results are impressive. Yet for many weight lifters, Crossfit, Pilates, and enthusiasts of other workout approaches, looking at the body from a relaxation and structural prospective can be threatening.

We can become myopic in our exercise. We get into one thing, work our asses off, see gains, and makes friends. Then the thought of bringing in another discipline feels heretical. We have invested so much in our sport that our cognitive dissonance compels us to resist anything different. When we look at the most successful athletes with the longest careers we often see more than the traditional training routine.

---

[57] http://www.rolf.org/about/research

Using Rolfing® to help recover from injuries, prevent injuries, and improve performance is taking the cross training model to the next level. Athletes learn that a myofascial system that is resilient, a structure that is aligned, and a body that is rejuvenated will naturally access their core muscles. This body will always perform better. In running, where it is easy to measure improvements, every runner who completed a series of ten sessions with me set a new personal record.

Are You Overwhelmed by Chronic Illness or Chronic Pain?

Have You Reached Your Last Resort?

As you're reading this, are you in pain? Have you done all the tests, had all the treatments, but you're still in pain? I'm not talking about that sprained ankle from your run yesterday; I mean that back pain or general malaise you've had for years.

According to the CDC, in 2005, 133 million Americans—almost one out of every two adults—had at least one chronic illness.[58] Your illness might affect your physical abilities, your appearance, or your independence. You may not be able to work, causing financial problems. About one-fourth of people with chronic conditions have one or more daily activities limited. For children, chronic pain and illness can be frightening because they may not understand why it is happening to them.

There is hope. Let's look at a few key facets to healing[59] a chronic condition.

Chronic vs. Acute

You injure yourself, you get a cold—that's acute pain or illness. Chronic illness or pain is the type that doesn't go away *or* keeps coming back.

---

[58] Centers for Disease Control and Prevention, Chronic Diseases and Health Promotion, http://www.cdc.gov/chronicdisease/overview/index.htm

[59] http://en.wikipedia.org/wiki/Alternative_medicine

According to the American Pain Foundation, more than 25% of Americans over 20 say they've experienced pain that lasted longer than 24 hours, and 42% have endured pain lasting longer than a year. Chronic pain costs the U.S. over $100 billion per year.[60]

Allopathic medicine, or standard medicine, is great at fixing trauma and killing infections. We are becoming bionic with all of the advances in surgery. Premature babies' survival rates continue to improve. Science and medicine keep on developing more technology as their contribution to healthcare.

Unfortunately, preventing and healing chronic illness and pain is not allopathic medicine's strong suit. Fixing an immediate problem is different than preventing or curing a long-term problem. Andrew Weil[61], MD, the Harvard-trained doc, internationally renowned author, and University of Arizona medical school professor, claims that "modern medicine" is not the place to go for healing chronic conditions. He directs his patients and medical fellows to look at holistic medicine.

Secondary Gains

Before we can explore using holistic medicine for healing chronic conditions, we need to look at some of the reasons we might have a stubborn condition. Sometimes the underlying explanation for the development of a particular problem is actually a secondary *gain*. (I'll explain that in a second.) For some people, these "other" reasons can sabotage even the best allopathic or holistic medicine.

What do I mean when I say you might *gain* from being sick? I'll use myself as an example: As a boy, when I was sick I got a lot of attention and I allowed myself to receive it. As an adult I certainly didn't consciously

---

[60] The American Academy of Pain Medicine Foundation - AAPM Facts and Figures on Pain, http://www.painmed.org/patientcenter/facts_on_pain.aspx

[61] http://www.drweil.com/

decide to get sick to get attention…but at some point, I realized that some small part of me enjoyed the upside of being sick.

I am not saying you're sick because you're seeking attention. I don't know anyone who does that. In fact, one of my clients, a work-at-home mom, told me the exact opposite: that when she's sick, it's the only time she doesn't feel guilty telling her kids she needs to rest quietly, ALONE, in her room! Yet, I have seen, with myself and others, that as kids we learned that when we needed attention, often the only available means was being sick.

Your first instinct is to survive not just physically but also emotionally. When the more positive options are unavailable, you default to the less advantageous options. Much of this occurs unconsciously. I once had a client—we'll call her Sue—who had "tried everything" to get well. Sue started with the medical docs, then moved on to holistic practitioners. She came to me desperate. We talked as she went through the Rolfing® SI process. Over the course of a few sessions, she revealed that her father had been domineering. Her mother was the "loving one." It soon became clear to her that she had unconsciously learned that in order to get attention she needed to be sick. Her father would back off and her mother would pour attention on her.

As a child in Sue's world, there was no other way to receive attention than to be sick. That wasn't true as an adult. Unfortunately, her body and mind were trained to get sick to get love. When she understood how her past was haunting her present and allowed herself to really feel the sadness she couldn't feel as a child, she got well. Knowledge will set you free. Usually you will also need to fully experience the feelings—from beginning to end—that you were not allowed to express. Then your new awareness can have its full effect.

Much of Sue's healing was letting go of her old story of always being sick. That meant she needed to let go of how she described herself as well as her way of relating to people as a sick person. She quit her support group because, as she described it, they were supporting the sickness. By letting go of her unconscious affinity for being sick, her holistic medicinal treatments worked. She got well.

Healing Chronic Pain

When you originally injured your back, for example, it may have caused your stomach, pelvis, and legs to become tighter—your body braced itself against the pain. You can take muscle relaxers, massage, and heat and ice your back, but if your body tightened up *around* the injury, the pain isn't going away. You may relax the sore back muscles, but the other tight muscles will pull everything awry and you'll be in pain again. Sometimes, people spend years bracing against pain, producing more tension and more pain than the original trauma.

A traumatic injury[62] or chronic pain produces stress. One of the biochemical effects of stress is that the body gets more physically tense, which causes more stress. Releasing chronic tension can be a huge aid in healing chronic pain.

Many holistic treatments focus on releasing the old tension and teaching the body-mind not to reproduce it. As you learn to relax, your body's instinctual bracing against the pain relaxes, diminishing your pain and allowing you to relax more. The vicious cycle of tension-to-pain is reversed.

For some of us, diet plays a huge part in treating pain. Just today I spoke to a client who told me that getting off of wheat and dairy eliminated his joint pain. As a bonus, he lost 25 pounds. Simple holistic solutions of changing behaviors and releasing stress transform chronic pain. Expand your healthcare options to the noninvasive practices of holistic medicine. Consider treatments that you haven't tried before. Rolfing® SI's focus on chronic tension makes it an excellent treatment for any chronic pain that is in part tied to your soft tissue, stress, and structure.

Get Out of the Box
Our thinking and our healthcare system are oriented toward fixing problems. Plus, things are so complicated and confusing these days,

---

[62] http://en.wikipedia.org/wiki/Injury

with all the tests and newly-identified illnesses, we have given away authority over our own bodies to the healthcare system. If you have good insurance, it almost seems like free healthcare—it often doesn't cost extra out-of-pocket for all the tests and specialists—but with that sense of healthcare entitlement, we gave up self-responsibility.

Getting well may mean doing more than what some expert tells you to do. Don't assume the expert knows everything; don't give up your body. You may need to seek out new information and new therapies. You likely will have to pay for these therapies. Like the athlete, you will need to invest in your body to be strong.

Get the Support You Need
As you step out of the institutional box of our healthcare system, you will need support. Do your due diligence, **become an expert about what you have.** Don't just look at what standard medicine and science says. Look for what others who had similar conditions did to get well. Who knows what you are going through better than someone who went through it too? Learn from their failures and successes. It's rarely one thing that gets a person well. There are no magic pills.

The Internet is a great place to start. People want to help. Many current or past sufferers become geeks about their illnesses. There are people out there who know a tremendous amount firsthand about their illness. Find out if they are still sick or if they are getting well. Discern which information is useful to you.

I am often amazed by my clients. Many will come to see me as an authority on their condition. I freely admit they know more about their illness than I do. They certainly know what doesn't work. Frequently they will comment that before they started their healing journey they had no interest in holistic medicine. After first trying all of the traditional means to get better, they found themselves trying holistic therapies and finally getting well.

A year ago I had a client, we'll call John, who was going from one specialist to another while continuing to get worse. After listening to his wife and his kids, John decided to see a naturopath in Seattle where he lived. The naturopath ran a few tests and came back with a new diagnosis which essentially described a nutritional imbalance, not the degenerative disease that he was diagnosed with previously. Within a month, he was feeling better. In six months his regular doc said his tests were normal and there was no need for the liver transplant he'd been told he would need.

John is now an evangelist for holistic health. His year of healing converted him into a champion of changing your lifestyle to get well. He no longer eats the foods that made him sick. When he was last in to see me, he shared that he can't understand why someone would not give up a few things to feel good.

The Downside of Getting Well

I always mention to my clients that getting well is like getting in shape. At first, it's work. It's not always (if ever) fun in the beginning. But stick with your program and you will see results. It gets easier—and then it becomes fun.

You know how, when you first start working out, you're actually more tired than normal and usually sore? Well, when you start on a program of holistic health, something similar can happen: as the stress leaves your body, so do the old toxins held in your tissue. These toxins can be from normal physiology such as uric and lactic acid from your body's metabolism. They can also be from chemicals or drugs you were exposed to. Twenty-five years ago I remember working on a big man who grew up applying chemical solvents. For several sessions the room reeked of those chemicals. It took several washings before the smell was gone from my hands. After several weeks the client was feeling better than he could recall ever feeling. My hands and the room stopped smelling.

One law of homeopathy, a holistic medical therapy, states that you get well in reverse order to how you got sick. That means that the more recent symptoms may show themselves as they release from your body, while the older symptoms might present themselves later. It is like peeling an onion one layer at a time. For many, getting well is just a matter of removing the tensions and toxins that created the illness or pain. For others, it will also involve rebalancing. It will involve work for everyone.

There Is More Than Hope

Over the last 30-plus years, I have treated thousands of clients, many referred to me by physicians. The one thing that is consistent with all these clients is their commitment to get well. Some come feeling desperate; others come because they just want to feel better. A few have freely admitted that they were as guilty as the next person when it came to not investing in their health. Often they admit they had been better at investing in the maintenance of their cars than their bodies.

Recognize that "chronic" means that the cause has existed for a long time. Explore any secondary reasons that might be a benefit from being sick. Expand your thinking and options by seeking the help you need. Get the support you need along the way and understand that getting well can have setbacks.

There are no panaceas, there is just collaboration. With the help of many practitioners, I have seen people cure themselves of "incurable" conditions. I cured myself of Asperger's Syndrome through my journey. At age 59, my body and my mind are doing things that I thought impossible when I was 19.

Chronic illness and pain can be transformed. It will take work and investment on your part. You are worth the effort. Create your support team and get started today. Please apply this strategy to your children. The rate of chronic health conditions among children in the United States increased from 12.8% in 1994 to 26.6% in 2006, according to results of a new study published in the *Journal of the American Medical Association*. Children respond very quickly to alternative therapies; we adults are a little tougher.

How Rolfing® SI Can Help RSD (Reflex Sympathetic Dystrophy) and Chronic Pain

RSD, as with many chronic pain conditions, can become debilitating. Blog Talk Radio interviewed me[63] on how Rolfing® can help treat RSD (Reflex Sympathetic Dystrophy[64]) and Chronic Pain.

Rolfing® SI's effectiveness with chronic pain comes from the release of chronic stress and tension that, even if it's not the cause of the pain, at least makes it worse. The fundamental stress of life can build, so that a little problem evolves into a major condition.

In the interview, I also explained how Mindfulness Stress Reduction and other holistic techniques can be very effective in dealing with chronic pain. Check out www.stressed.org for more on how mindfulness Stress Reduction[65] can help.

The Truth about Your Muscles

Do your muscles hurt? Do they not serve you like they used to? Are they not toned like you want? Do you have frequent muscle injuries—or muscles that are not performing like they should? Is your once strong and supple body now less strong, and tighter? Do you feel old? Do you work out regularly, doing what you were taught was the way to work out? Don't blame your muscles.

The Problem

You'll probably be surprised to hear this, but the problem didn't start with your muscles; it started as a movement problem. You can have

---

[63] http://www.blogtalkradio.com/thematrix777/2010/06/04/living-with-rsd-reflex-sympathetic-dystrophy

[64] http://en.wikipedia.org/wiki/Complex_regional_pain_syndrome

[65] http://en.wikipedia.org/wiki/Mindfulness-based_stress_reduction

stronger, more resilient and better-toned muscles if you give them what they need. To do that you need to understand the first rule of muscles: when a muscle does a job it's meant to do, it gets stronger, more resilient, and sometimes bigger. When a muscle does a job it's not meant to do, it's a micro-trauma to the muscle. We all know a major trauma will produce scar tissue. Well, the same is true with the micro-traumas from muscle misuse.

Those micro-traumas produce scar tissue over time, and eventually the fascia in and around the muscle goes from spandex to dried leather.

A subtle, gradual strain can have a cumulative effect that is as great as a major trauma. A "stress fracture" may sound like a minor injury, but is still a fracture in a bone. Over time your body creates more scar tissue (fascia) to help protect, heal, and assist the injured area. Because the injury is so gradual, we don't realize what's happening until it is an injury, then we blame it on aging. It's not just aging, though; over time, you produced the same effect that an injury produces instantaneously. This is, in part, due to the fact that increased tension produces decreased awareness. What comes to your awareness is not the gradual scarring; what comes to your attention is the resulting injury. The scarring not only restricts movement, it restricts circulation furthering the muscle's decline. The injury that seems to develop out of the blue and won't go away is not like a specific injury caused by one event. Because it built up over weeks, months, or even years, the injury doesn't go away like a bruise would. It has layers of scar tissue and often involves whole-body compensational patterns.

The Solution: Transforming Your Muscles

Fixing the problem requires understanding the cause. When a muscle or any body part repeatedly does a job it's not primarily designed to do, it becomes a micro-trauma. It's easy to understand that when we walk or run, our legs are meant to track straight. In other words our knees should be pointing forward. So you can imagine how years of a leg rotated out would produce a chronic injury someplace in your body—probably many places in that instance.

Owen Marcus

Unfortunately, pulling or strengthening the body part back into alignment is, at best, only temporary. In the long run it can cause more problems because you are adding more strain on top of a chronic strain pattern. You need to release the strain, realign the body part, and learn the natural, correct way to move that body part and its muscles.

The easiest way to think about this is to think about what primitive man did with his body. He walked and ran. He didn't walk or run sideways. Yes, those muscles can do that, but you can imagine how your legs would feel if that were the only way you propelled yourself.

The bottom line: **When a muscle does a job it is not meant to do, it gets tighter. When a muscle does a job it is meant to do, it gets stronger.** We've been trained to believe that a hard, tight muscle is a strong muscle. To the amazement of many of my 'hard and tight' male clients, relaxed or supple muscles and fascia always produced better results. I had men who stopped lifting for a month to receive four sessions and rest their bodies. When they went back they were stronger. If you aren't getting stronger, look at how you are using your body.

The good news is that you can reverse this process by releasing the scar tissue, using the muscles as they were designed to be used, and making sure your body receives the necessary nutrition. The release can be done through yoga, massage, and Rolfing® SI. Yoga and massage are excellent for the more recent restrictions, while Rolfing® SI addresses the chronic issues.

Over the years, I've treated many Olympic and professional athletes. Originally I presumed that they would not be mal-trained or over-trained. I was wrong. Even today they tell me that most of their training is archaic, still following the old models that produce injuries. Beliefs such as "the more the better," "no pain no gain," and "fast and hard" continue to tighten and injure muscles.

My Super Slow workouts with the Exercise Institute based on the work of Doug McGuff, MD[66] have not only made me stronger than ever, they have loosened me up. Rather than fast reps or many reps, you do a few very slowly. Those movements, much like my Natural Running™ form, mimic what our muscles were designed to do. Given that our genome is 99.9% the same as it was 2.5 million years ago, following movement patterns adapted from what our ancestors did is good for us. Running correctly, lifting weights correctly, and exercise that mimics natural movements are the best gifts you can give your muscles.

Are Your Bones Holding You Up?

In spite of what we were taught, our bones are not meant to hold us up. Think about it, your vertebral discs are like the jelly in a jelly donut— they are spacers that allow your back to bend. When your abdominal and low back muscles become tight and short, you lose your waist. Those jelly donuts become pancakes as your back compresses, then your spine attempts to support you. Until then, the small muscles and ligaments of the back acted as a suspension system, much like a suspension bridge[67], where the cables are holding the bridge up.

The long bones of the body, such as the thigh bones (femur), are also not meant to be the sole source of support. As with the back, when the femur takes too much of the load, you see stress in the hip joints and knees. For years, I have seen dozens of runners wear out their knees because of compression and misalignment. Don't get me wrong, I think the human body is meant to run. We just need to do it as we are meant to do it.

---

[66] http://www.bodybyscience.net/home.html/

[67] http://en.wikipedia.org/wiki/Suspension_bridge

In his book, *Body by Science*[68], Doug McGuff, MD, the leading expert on intense exercise, quotes a study by Manohoar Pahjabi. In the journal *Spine,* Pahjabi explains how the spine itself can't support a small load. It needs the soft tissue[69] (muscles and fascia) of the entire trunk to support the load.

In the last decade, we've heard a lot of talk about 'core strength.' We Rolfers™ were speaking about core muscles forty years ago. We all agree that we are more powerful and less injury prone when we move and work from our core. I often see patients who were told strengthening their core would help their back. In theory this is true. The problem lies with its application. An abdominal soft tissue system and back muscle system that is tight and short will feel better at first. Quickly, however, they will grow ever tighter and shorter.

When the soft tissue is relaxed, then strengthening the core occurs without tightening and shortening. The back and its big muscles don't become a brace that holds you up. They are there to move you, not to be posture muscles.

How to Have Your Soft Tissue Take the Load

Beyond stretching, you need to release the restrictions. If the soft tissue hasn't turned into leather, stretching can often create the lengthening and relaxation. Yet, the people who need to decompress the most often find stretching to be frustrating.

Rolfing® can begin the reversal. I repeatedly have clients, within a month, come in to tell me they are taller from the decompression of the soft tissue.

---

[68] http://www.amazon.com/Body-Science-Research-Strength-Training/dp/0071597174

[69] http://en.wikipedia.org/wiki/Soft_tissue

Sports Performance Enhancement

How do you improve your performance without drugs? Tune your number one instrument: your body.

Men in particular will not hesitate to spend money for the newest development in equipment technology. We covet a new set of skies, clubs, or maybe that new mountain bike. We like our toys. But how often do you consider the next advancement in improving your bodies? About the only time any of us do anything for our bodies is when we have to—when something breaks down.

Your Body Is More Than the Sum of Its Parts

Your body is your most important piece of equipment. No matter how good your clubs, skis, or shoes are, if your body is not performing at its peak level, you won't get the results you want. Chances are you also won't be having as much fun. For a while you might be able to push it, but eventually your body will tire.

Several years ago, I conducted the first study on Rolfing® and sports performance with Arizona State University (ASU). We ran three groups of elite runners through; only one group received Rolfing®. The intent was to quantify the improvements the runners experienced from the Rolfing®. To do that, the researchers decided to reduce the body's performance down to small mechanical movements and measure those. Shank angle (the angle of the ankle relative to the knee) was one such measurement. These measurements changed little, yet each Rolfing subject's injuries disappeared and they all set new personal records.

Rolfing® puts into practice the principle that the whole is much greater than the sum of its parts. Yes, most clients come to see us because they have a specific problem. But to fix the problem, increase performance significantly, and sustain those improvements, we need to look beyond the parts.

As you play a sport, your body is dealing with many variables, including gravity, coordination, strength, aerobic capacity, endurance, and structural alignment. Each of these factors has many interrelated aspects constantly affecting your performance. Your bad knee could come from your rotated femur, which comes from the shortness in your piriformis and gracillis muscles, which may have first started shortening because of your everted foot (a foot turned out).

To deal with all the primary and secondary causes that limit your performance, you must address your entire body. You need to release and re-organize your fascia. This thin connective tissue holds everything together. Over the years it may become distorted, causing you to feel like you were performing in a suit that's a size too small. Because the process of distortion was slow, you are only aware of the problems—sore back, aching knees, etc.—you may not even notice your hindered performance and just chalk it up to aging.

Most clients come to me to alleviate a problem. That's the easy part. Transforming the entire suit is the challenge I love. After releasing, the pain is gone and the client invariably starts to experience gradual improvements in performance. They are amazed how much better they are performing—they hadn't realized the full impact of their restrictions.

Last year a man in his fifties came to me after a life of playing many sports and the usual associated injuries. He was hoping to avoid shoulder surgery. Before he finished his tenth session, his shoulder was 95% better, his performance in each of his sports was better and easier than it had been in decades. But the most exciting effect was that he was having more fun. He said he felt like a kid again.

Learn Not to Recreate the Problems

After their bodies begin to loosen and straighten, I start to teach my clients what I call the *Natural Walk*. This way of walking goes against what most of us do: leaning back as we walk causing us to fight gravity. I teach clients how to use gravity to do most the work. For sports like skiing and running, this is huge. Even for sports such as swimming and cycling, I see improvements because clients learn to use their core muscles correctly. When you get this walk down, you click into using your body as it was designed to be used. Using gravity and your core muscles correctly gives you an enormous advantage.

When your fascial suit loosens, becomes flexible, and straightens, your range of motion, recovery time, and adaptability significantly improve. Your newly resilient body feels younger as your soft tissue deeply relaxes.

Your breathing also improves because your chest, diaphragm and back are looser. While in Scottsdale, Olympic runners I worked on told to me that the biggest benefit from their Rolfing® was not the healing of their injuries, rather it was their increased vital capacity (the ability to exchange air).

Improving performance is more than just getting stronger, becoming more flexible, getting better trained, or upgrading equipment, it is transforming your entire structure. This magnitude of change often seems unrealistic until you experience it. I certainly wouldn't have believed that, at age 59, I would be one inch taller, a lot faster and looser, and better coordinated than I was at 19. Our bodies are constantly changing. Fortunately, we get to decide *how* they change.

Are You at Risk of Tearing Your Achilles Tendon?

If your calf is tight, you could be one of the half-million people who tear their Achilles tendon every year. For many people, it means the tendon snaps off at its attachment to the heel. As anyone who went through that experience will tell you, it is excruciatingly painful.

While it's the most common tendon tear, Achilles tendon tears are preventable simply by keeping the muscles that pull on the tendon loose, elastic, and long. Many years ago when I had my holistic medical clinic in Scottsdale, an office manager for an orthopedic surgeon sent her surgeon to me because he wasn't healing from his torn Achilles tendon. Also, she needed him to relax—or she was going to quit!

This doctor was a nice guy who was very tense. He admitted that he didn't follow his own advice and went back to work too soon after his first tear. He ended up snapping the tendon off the bone a second time. After watching the general stiffness of his body as he moved and feeling the hardness of his tissue, I mentioned that he was tense. He quickly retorted, "No, I'm not tense. I just have muscular anomalies."

Every time I lightly touched a new area he felt pain prompting him to give me a new diagnosis. After several minutes of this, I stopped working and told him point-blank: "Unless you learn to relax, you are not going to improve." I explained to him that his tension was systemic, it wasn't just his calf. His general tension and restricted movement pattern had allowed his calf to become so badly tense and his tendon so brittle that when he tore it the first time all he had done was turn the corner in his office. That's right: while walking around a corner, his tendon snapped off the bone again.

How to Prevent Achilles Tears

These tendons don't tear unless the calf muscles they attach to pull so hard they cause the tendon to tear or even snap off of the heel. Lower leg muscles develop their tightness and shortness from years of never fully extending them. You wouldn't do bicep curls and only extend your arm out halfway, because you know the bicep would eventually shorten. That's what happened with the calf because of how these clients walked—they never extended the heel behind them. It is as if they are wearing high heels, shortening the calf muscles with every step. (See section on the *Natural Walk* later in the book for more explanation.)

Stretching and massage are great at keeping the calves loose, but they can't counter years of a poor stride that never stretches them out. After a few decades of the muscles and connective tissues tightening and shortening, many people require remedial therapies such as Rolfing® SI to regain the elasticity and length.

If you find your calves feel tight when you try to extend them, get some work done on them! It's much easier to prevent an Achilles tear than to recover from one.

How to Heal Your Old Sprains and Strains

Do you have an old sprain (over stretched ligament), an old strain (torn muscle, tendon, or ligament), or a bad ankle that you injured with a wrong turn?

With the traditional *R.I.C.E.* treatment (rest, ice, compress, and elevate), your immediate pain and swelling eventually dissipates, then you slowly start reusing your injured joint—knowing it could happen all over again with the wrong move. But that's just managing the pain; it's not healing an injury.

The Problem

So what do you do with that bad ankle you keep spraining? You've probably tried stretching and exercise, and it might have helped for a while. Taking anti-inflammatories, muscle relaxers, and pain pills manage your discomfort, but aren't solving the problem. Your doc tells you surgery is not an option, which is actually a relief. So what IS the solution?

To really fix it, and have it stay fixed, you need to treat the causes. First, you need to "fix" your soft tissue—muscles, tendons, ligaments, and fascia. At some point, after the first injury and a little more each time, your soft tissue became encased in scar tissue. This is only because your body did what it should do: it sent fibroblasts, "the mending cells," to the injured area to weld together and support the injury. But once the injury healed, the body's natural cast did not dissolve away as it might have when you were a child. Now you're stuck with this connective tissue "cast" after you're well.

Additionally, while you're limping around and protecting the injury, other parts of your body tighten up, and you develop bad habits in your movement. For instance, using the other leg and twisting not to hurt the injured ankle creates a structural and behavioral pattern that, in the end, can be worse than the original injury. Parts of your body are tense and distorted, while other parts are structurally weak and vulnerable. Now you're an injury waiting to happen.

The Solution

Complete healing must involve releasing the fascial (scar tissue) adhesions. That "cast" your body didn't dissolve has to be manually dissolved. Feel the ankle you keep spraining, and compare it to the one that is relatively normal. The bad ankle is less moveable and thicker. This thick and hard tissue should be thin, subtle, and fluid. The tendons of the foot coming from the muscles in the lower leg should slide through your ankle. Your thick, tight band prevents natural movement.

Rolfing® SI will slowly release this band. It's amazing to feel in just a few minutes of work how much movement is possible. It'll feel like you took off the steel band and oiled the cables running through your ankle. Once it's released, circulation and elasticity also increases, helping you heal even faster.

The more challenging work is the re-aligning of the body after years of compensating. Once everything is released, we need to re-organize your whole body—that's where Rolfing® SI goes beyond other therapies. There are many therapies that infer or come out and state that they produce the same results as Rolfing® SI. While they may get some of the release, they don't organize the entire body around the gravitational line. Being relaxed is a huge improvement for many. To sustain that relaxation, let alone have it continue to improve, the body needs to be aligned.

A building that is not aligned will not last as long as its neighbor that is. Nor will an athlete who moves in an inefficient manner avoid injury or outperform her competitors. A Rolfer™ is a human architect making sure all your parts are where they should be. Our goal is to get the most change possible throughout your structure and have it last—so you don't keep coming back.

Often, a secondary problem—indirectly caused by the original injury—is what brings a client to me. You might come in complaining of a worsening back problem. As I watch you walk and ask you questions, we may figure out that your back problems started after you sprained your ankle. Your normal walk now has a subtle limp that gradually caused other problems. Others could see it, but it felt normal to you because you adapted so well. You'll need to unlearn that limp. You can fix the ankle, you can align the body, but you still need to re-educate the body.

After the re-alignment, your ankle will be less susceptible to injury and so will the rest of your body. While in Scottsdale, I treated many world-class runners who continued to sprain their ankles. It was amazing to hear these runners talk about how accustomed they became to the slow process of tightening. When their ankle and its related problems healed, their performance went to a new level—every time, with every client.

I have a 37-year-old client right now who is training for a half-marathon. She had sprained knees, sprained ankles, and terrible movement habits. But after a few Rolfing® SI sessions, she told me, "I run better and faster than I did when I was 18!" Everybody performs better after releasing the old scar tissue. We often don't know what we lost until we get it back.

Loose joints are a common problem that is exacerbated by sports. The unstable joint may be hyper-mobile, meaning it moves too much. For example, a knee may extend back where it causes the whole leg to bow. For most people this doesn't present a problem, but you can imagine the stress that knee would experience training for a marathon. With ankles you may have a joint that is too mobile in one direction. Here that joint continues to become more vulnerable to sprains. Invariably above and below the hyper-mobile joint is restricted and misaligned soft tissue.

Once restriction is released and organized, the loose joint gradually tightens up. The lack of support shifts to a feeling of a stable structure. The reinjuring and the strain on the ligaments stop. The uneven or ex-cessive wear on the cartilage can also stop. There are times when the structural reorganizing exceeded expectations, yet the severity of the damage to the joint requires surgery for that joint to function properly.

Tune Your Body for Skiing

A lot of us believe that the secret to better skiing is better equipment. Let's face it—the sport equipment companies are very convincing. So we spend hundreds of dollars getting top-of-the-line equipment, we dream of strapping it on and taking that great run.

But to ensure a great ski season, there's one vital piece of equipment: your body. Even with all your state-of-the-art equipment, you need your body to be at its peak. Your body needs to be more than strong; it needs to be loose, aligned, and relaxed to assure top performance.

What Others Don't Tell You

Life just seems to happen, right? You wake up one morning stiff, tired, and sore after a hard day on the slopes. It's like your body is saying, "Hey! Newsflash! You're not young anymore!" What happened to that body that could ski all weekend and play all night?

We blame age, but that's not it. We do lose our edge over time, but that's because of stress, injuries, bad habits, years of hard work, maybe some minor accidents, never stretching—this all causes your body to gradually tighten and misalign. And that's why you wake up stiff, sore, and feeling battered.

But here's the secret: the inherent gifts of childhood—suppleness, strength, natural alignment—are recoverable, and even upgradable.

Upgrade Your Body

Over time, every stress—even minor incidents, like occasional back pain—produces scar tissue. If you were a butcher, you would call this gristle. And it increasingly restricts your body's movement. As your body tightens, it causes misalignment. A tight and misaligned body cannot perform as well as it did with the suppleness of youth, which explains that stiff, sore, battered feeling.

You may have tried stretching, or some kind of bodywork therapy, only to be more frustrated with your body. But the problem could be that your soft tissue is now solid gristle. To get a body that can truly stretch, many people need remedial help.

The Solution – The Secret to Sustainable Peak Performance

If you want a different result, try a different solution. To convert that gristle back to soft tissue, you must release it. Yes, it will release. Meat can be tenderized and your tight soft tissue can become resilient again. With slow pressure, the gristly connective tissue fibers in and around your muscles can become supple again. The bio-chemical change in the fiber comes, in part, from increased circulation. As the circulation and movement increases, the once self-perpetuating tightening process reverses, and your increased movement loosens your tissue even more.

Everything from a good massage to very specific assisted stretching can move you in this direction. The fast trackers will often see me for Rolfing® SI. When I was working with Olympic athletes and professional ball players, we did a study with Arizona State University on elite runners. Every Rolfing® SI subject alleviated his/her injuries and set new personal records. The body is amazing in its ability to regenerate. It only needs a little help.

Over the years, we have grown to see the importance of stretching, rest, core strength (as Rolfers™, we were promoting all of this 30 years ago), and our mind's attitude as critical to increasing our performance and pleasure. The remaining question is: What do we do about our past sins? All of the above will be limited if our bodies are tight and misaligned. To achieve the most from these activities and our bodies, we need to reverse the years of stress.

Your Best Investment

Invest in your most important equipment—your body. The risk is low and the potential gain is high. Not only can your old injuries improve or disappear, but you may also find that you have the ease and joy of a child's body once again. I would be as happy to speak to you about your options as I would be to work with you. But whatever you do, I suggest you step out of the traditional box to get nontraditional results.

The Secret to the Body You Want

We spend **over $80 Billion** a year on diets. That is the same amount we spent annually on the Iraq War.

Why are you losing the war on fat? Because we don't deal with the underlying cause: stress.

Stress causes your body to crave quick energy carbohydrates. Stress also shuts down the parasympathetic nervous system[70], thereby shutting down full digestive function. Most destructively, stress puts you in a survival response of reacting to what's in front of you, causing you to forget all your commitments.

It Gets Worse

Chronic stress becomes a learned state reinforced by the soft tissue tension in your body. Much like a lab rat, you reinforce the stress response[71] while anchoring it in your fascial system (the connective tissue that holds everything together and the organ of stress). As you continue to wind yourself tighter, you continue to gain weight. The latest fad diet works for a while, but deprivation only enhances the survival response.

A Simple Solution

Trying to get rid of stress in your life never works. It is impossible to be completely unstressed. The two secrets are: unlearning the stress response, and removing the chronic stress[72], which perpetuates the stress, from your body.

---

[70] http://en.wikipedia.org/wiki/Parasympathetic_nervous_system

[71] http://en.wikipedia.org/wiki/Fight-or-flight_response

[72] http://en.wikipedia.org/wiki/Chronic_stress

You learned to adapt to the stress/survival response as your default state. You can unlearn it. Back in the mid-1990s at my Scottsdale Institute for Health and Medicine we taught Jon Kabat-Zinn, Ph.D's, Mindfulness Stress Reduction Program. People didn't come to us to lose weight, but when they learned how to make relaxation their default state, gentle weight loss was often a consequence.

Over the years of treating thousands of clients through Rolfing® SI for all variations of stress, I have seen hundreds lose weight they had previously struggled with—once they lost their chronic stress. Good bodywork removes chronic stress and teaches the body-mind when not to go into a stress response.

What Is the Problem with Cellulite?

When I had my clinic, strings of women saw me for Rolfing® SI for one reason: cellulite. They'd tried everything to eliminate their cellulite. They did the exercise, diet, and creams to no avail. Sometimes a woman would come to me for a usual Rolfing® SI problem, such as back pain. Six months later, her cellulite was completely gone. Then her friends were asking what her secret was.

Losing the cellulite was rarely an immediate effect; it usually occurred months later. As a client's body continued to relax, the body's physiology got the message that it didn't need to store fat for the ever-present survival response. Their bodies increased circulation from better movement patterns and slowly burned away the old fat.

If you read up on cellulite, you'll learn that fascia, that thin connective tissue that Certified Rolfers™ release, is what holds the fat that creates the cellulite. If the fascia remains tight and thick, the fat can't burn away.

How Does Rolfing® SI Dissolve Cellulite?

How is it possible that several Rolfing® SI sessions and a few months of integrating the change can remove cellulite from the hips and thighs when nothing else did? The fascia along the outside of the leg becomes scar tissue from the stress, or I as call it, micro-traumas, over the years. Intended to be much like spandex, the fascia instead becomes like dried leather. This leather not only loses its elasticity, it also becomes impermeable to proper fluid exchange.

In the course of the series of Rolfing® SI sessions, the tight fascia of the legs release and so do the stress patterns that created it.

One stress pattern is how the legs are used. I have yet to see a client who walked properly. Even the Olympic runners I treated were out of balance with their walk. Because of the imbalance, the extra strain on the soft tissue of the outer leg eventually creates the scar tissue, setting up the cellulite. Additionally, other sets of muscles and fascial sheets are not used as they were intended to be used due to the misalignment.

Releasing the tissue increases circulation. Realignment and learning the *Natural Walk* decreases the strain pattern while toning underused muscles. For example, women will come back after a few sessions amazed they have a butt when they never had one. They ask how that could happen. It happens because the gluteal (butt) muscles are now in a position to be used.

By removing the cause, the body will normally remove the effects—the cellulite. Your good diet and exercise then start having the effects they should. Cellulite is not inevitable; it is a consequence of stress, structural imbalance, and movement imbalance, along with diet.

Reverse Aging

"John" was a plastic surgeon and client who became a friend of mine, and we used to debate why Rolfing® SI was helping him. He claimed that fascia couldn't change, so I said, "Then you tell me why your chronic back pain is gone and your golf game is the best it's ever been."

John didn't like working on patients who weren't healthy; their fascia was dried out and not elastic, and they didn't respond well. We did agree that fascia is like tree rings: you can tell the relative age of a body by the quality of the fascia. Resilient fascia responds well to plastic surgery, Rolfing® SI, and, I would argue, all healthcare interventions.

What Occurs with Aging

We've resigned ourselves to having our bodies tighten, slouch, and dry out as we get older. But I've had clients in their 80's who were healthy, happy, and active with a posture and walk you would expect in a younger person. Their "fascial suit" hadn't shrunk as it had for their peers. If the tissue that holds everything together is thin, resilient, and subtle, the muscles and organs will be too.

How to Reverse Aging

First, decrease the stressors that damage your health. Is your diet contributing to or sabotaging your health? What is producing tension in your life? Remove or decrease those emotional stressors and you can change your life. There are certainly stressors that we can't remove. Yet we can learn to change our response to them. It is much easier for a relaxed body to learn to let go of a stress response.

When I had a stress reduction business, I discovered that we learn to be tense and we can learn to relax! You taught your body the stress response[73] that produces the tension which contributes to aging. Replace your stress response with a stress *release* response. You will feel younger and look younger.

Be proactive: detox your body of old environmental and diet toxins. Detox your body of the chronic stress through bodywork and Rolfing®. Then focus on maintenance and prevention. Do yoga, get out for walks,

---

[73] http://en.wikipedia.org/wiki/Fight-or-flight_response

get daily exercise, and learn to eat organic foods. Increase the quality of your life. Do research on what works—not on fads, but on what makes you healthy. Find experts or therapists to assist you. You can reverse the effects of aging and slow the process down considerably.

Getting old is not an inevitability. Will you go gray and get wrinkles? Sure. Do you have to spend your later years immobile and in pain? NO. Going beyond prevention to rejuvenation is easy and fun with all the holistic therapies available. Live dangerously: try one.

Fascia is the organ of stress and aging

The father of stress research and the author of *Stress of Life*, Hans Selye[74], MD, stated "the beginning of the disease process starts with posture distortion." He went on to say that fascia, the connective tissue that holds our muscles, organs, and essentially the entire body together, is the organ system that becomes the organ of stress.

As stress and trauma accumulate in your body and in your life, your posture is inevitably affected by the tightness that stress and trauma cause. It's as if your "fascial suit" shrinks, causing your skeleton and posture to distort. A body that felt young and moved with grace becomes one that feels old and moves with limitations. Inside that body, your organs' functions are diminishing because of the structural restrictions.

Staying Young

This article[75] on Dr. Mercola's website[76] explains part of what I have seen in my body and that of hundreds of clients. As a Certified Rolfer™, I

---

[74] http://en.wikipedia.org/wiki/Hans_Selye

[75] http://articles.mercola.com/sites/articles/archive/2011/06/19/innovative-revolutionary-program-to-keep-your-body-biologically-oung.aspx?SetFocus=commentfocus&ShowAllComments= true#commentfocus

see that when the myofascial system scar tissue is released or broken down, the body becomes younger—much like the proper exercise program described in the article.

Fascia, as the organ of stress and aging, creates more of itself to cope with the chronic effects of over-eating, over-exercising and an overabundance of stress. One way the negative effects of these behaviors can be reversed is through Rolfing® SI.

The many men and women I convinced to cut back on exercise and increase animal protein consumption (these people were usually not consuming any) ended up with a younger body than they ever thought possible. We are trained to overdo everything. It is hard for some to cut back and make these life changes, particularly us driven men.

The Importance of Protein

When I first heard back in the 1970s that Dr. Rolf would often refuse to treat vegetarians, I thought she was being rigid. I quickly learned that she was being fair.

Many long term vegetarian clients I treated lack soft tissue tonicity. I remember one 40-year-old woman who was sent to me twenty-five years ago. As with all my clients, I liked her and wanted to do my best to help her get well. Looking at her body, I could see that she had no tone. This was confirmed when she laid down on the table. It was as if her soft tissue was a loose sack of melted Jell-O. Her tissue fell off her bones as she lay on the table. When I went to manipulate the tissue, it felt like melted Jell-O. There was nothing to push up against.

My first question was, "Are you a vegetarian?" She immediately responded with pride as she said, "I haven't eaten meat in twenty years."

---

[76] http://articles.mercola.com/members/Dr.-Mercola/default.aspx

I told her I felt she was unhealthy because she had no "meat on her bones." There was nothing to Rolf™.

I told her without animal protein she would not have any real muscles or connective tissue. I explained how many of her symptoms—low energy, chronic aches and pains, and joint injuries—could be traced back to her protein deficiencies. When I finished saying that I wouldn't continue to take her through the Rolfing® SI series of sessions, she got upset.

She insisted that I work on her. I assured her that I would if I could, but that without protein in her tissue there was nothing to work on. We had a dilemma: she wouldn't eat meat (or fish, poultry, or eggs) and I wouldn't treat her.

I explained that I wanted to help her. I also told her that I felt she was healthy except for her lack of protein. She listened when I explained that the lack of animal protein was causing her to age prematurely. From her increased wrinkling, worn joints, low life force energy, and collapsed posture, she looked and felt older than she was.

Unfortunately, my pitch to eat protein didn't inspire her. I never saw her again.

Particularly when I operated my clinic in Scottsdale, a good 20% of my female clients were protein deficient. Fortunately, not as much as this previous client—yet in every case when these clients would eat even a little animal protein we saw improvements in the tissue, structure, and health. In all honesty, some of the change they attributed to Rolfing® SI was actually from eating meat.

Our body is only as young as its connective tissue. Our connective tissue's youthfulness is dependent upon what we feed it and how we treat it. Again, stress makes it old. Rolfing® SI can reverse the chronic stress and its effect on the body. Applying the new body awareness that comes from Rolfing® SI will help keep the stress out of your body. Eating a diet that feeds the connective tissue will also keep you young, as will proper exercise.

Rolfing® SI focuses on releasing the chronic stress held in the fascia to align the body. As new fascial research is proving, the fascial system of the body is a huge, interconnected web. For example, a leg injury can set up back and abdominal strain. Recently, I saw a client because she had gotten an infection in her big toe; she walked off-kilter for days and ended up with back and neck pain.

More than 20 years ago, I took one of the first classes the French physician Jean-Pierre Barral, DO, taught to Certified Rolfers™, physical therapists, and physicians. His patients and the subsequent research proved that an organ which has a structural or fascial restriction will not perform at its highest level. Just as a scar on skin reduces its elasticity, fascial tightness constricts an organ's function.

You Are Only As Young As Your Structure

When you think of old, what do you think of? I suspect It's an elderly person, hunched over, walking slowly. Is that where you're headed? Before we explore how to avoid "getting old," let an expert explain why those older people are so hunched over:

> Some individuals may perceive their losing fight with gravity as a sharp pain in their back, others as the unflattering contour of their body, others as constant fatigue, yet others as an unrelentingly threatening environment. Those over forty may call it old age. And yet all these signals may be pointing to a single problem so prominent in their own structure, as well as others, that it has been ignored: they are off balance, they are at war with gravity. *Ida P. Rolf, Ph.D.*

The loss of structural integrity doesn't occur overnight. It takes decades of stress, poor posture, injuries, and repetitive motions to tighten the fascial suit your body wears. Much like an out-of-alignment building is more likely to collapse, so is a body. Research shows that "aging of the facial structures is attributed primarily to gravity."[77] As you know, once you enter the war of gravity, you will lose.

Years ago, I had a client in her eighties. Her complaint was that she had become an "old woman." I told her she was too young to be an old woman. She used to like to walk, but now walking was an act of courage. She wanted to stop walking as though she were always walking on ice. After the course of ten Rolfing® SI sessions, she was standing erect and walking normally again. It turned out an old injury in her twenties was the setup for her structural misalignment in her eighties. The most challenging part of the work was for her to unlearn the old protective walk she had developed. She was a good student; she continued to practice the Natural Walk technique, and it transformed her walk.

As most people age, they lose the ability to move sideways, bend, twist, and move quickly. Tension, structural collapse, and decreased muscle strength compound to make them old. The worse all this gets, the more the body and mind orient around survival rather than joy. As we all know, being afraid makes us tense.

Researchers and clinicians have developed simple procedures to test your relative structural age. The first is measuring how long and fast your gait is. The second, how quickly you can raise yourself form sitting on the floor, and how much you need to use your arms. The third set is your quality of movement—your range of movement, alignment (legs tracking straight), and coordination (balance and efficient movement). The next two weeks we will explore more of the causes and simple solutions for "old age."

---

[77] "Structural Aging: The Facial Recurve Concept. - PubMed - NCBI." Accessed December 7, 2014. http://www.ncbi.nlm.nih.gov/pubmed/17380358.

Misconceptions

"It's inevitable," we are told, "you shrink as you age." Well, two years after getting Rolfed at age 23, I was an inch taller. Now at 62, I'm an additional quarter of an inch taller. If you buy into limiting beliefs about your health, you create self-fulfilling prophecies. Or course, it takes more than having an empowering belief; it takes non-traditional action to produce extraordinary results.

What are some other assumptions we adopt that limit us that are not true?

A huge one is, "My genes determine my health." The new science of epigenetics teaches us that our response to our environment turns on or off our genes. The Human Genome Project discovered genetics are only responsible for about 10%of human disease.[78]

Another common belief, "I can't heal my chronic pain through diet change." The leading-edge research on how eating carbohydrates produce body fat and lead to inflammation – two principal causes of death – shows us how this simple change can produce considerable results. For years my clients lost significant weight, resolved chronic pain issues, and increased vitality by eliminating grains from their diet while making sure they were consuming enough high-quality meat.

"The body I have, I got from my parents, and I'm stuck with it." We are told that our genes predetermine our structure. Structure deterioration is expected – your feet will get flatter, your legs more bowed, your back stiffer, and your neck more forward. But just as my body continues to lengthen from the bodywork I receive, so can your body evolve out of its chronic difficulties.

Stress and environmental toxins cause our soft tissue to contract and deform, misaligning our skeleton. We treat the symptoms, or we can

---

[78] http://www.cdc.gov/niosh/topics/exposome/

back up and treat the underlying causes. We are taught not to question what is causing a condition; we are encouraged to get a drug to suppress the immediate symptom. When the condition keeps returning, it serves us to look at what is reproducing it and finding a sustainable remedy.

Not shrinking, keeping your weight down, healing your back pain, and feeling good as you age is possible when you step beyond our prevailing mindset of what it is to get old. When you are willing to explore holistic therapies and a healthy lifestyle your body can transform. I have clients in their 80s who are healthier than people half their age. More importantly, they feel young and vibrant.

How Your Structure Ages You

Your gait speed and variability predicts mortality.[79] As you slump over and walk slower, you shorten your life, or at least the quality of it. The progressive structural decline sets up many of these issues:

- slumped stance and height loss

- tendency to scoliosis and kyphosis (curving of the spine)

- belly extruding out

- rotation in legs and flatter feet

- plantar fasciitis and hammer toes

- turning non-posture muscles into posture-holding muscles with tightening and shortening of the muscles

---

[79] "Predicting Impending Death: Inconsistency in Speed Is a Selective and Early Marker." Accessed December 9, 2014.
http://www.ncbi.nlm.nih.gov/pmc/articles/PMC2562863/.

- loss of muscle tone

- fascial dehydrations and contraction (fascia holds the body to-gether and gives skin its shape) fascia's primary protein, colla-gen is injected into sagging skin, in attempts to bring back youth

- compression and misalignment of joints from unintended strain leads to: hip replacements, disc bulging, and osteoarthritis

For most of us, it's the little things that add up to age our structure, starting with sitting all day. "Studies have shown long periods of sitting is bad for the elderly, drastically increases your risk of cancer, and now new research confirms that being a couch potato at work is hazardous to your heart's health."[80] Then there is looking down at a screen for hours a day, which locks your head forward with no side movement. Your body is not different from our ancestors' bodies. Our ancestors were always moving and looking in all directions. Rather than being like a cat that can move in any direction at any moment, we adapt by devel-oping a protective posture. We become frozen prey.

Your footwear, often designed to support you, causes your foot struc-ture to become lazy and weak. This adds to adopting an unnatural stride. Kids just move; as adults we let our environment determine how we should move. Ergonomics is helping us get out of the behavior set of conforming to our furniture, but we still don't move enough.

All this sets your tight body up for more falls and the need for more sur-geries on your hips, knees, etc. With half of all hip surgeries leading to death, you may do best to avoid more than falling—avoid being brittle. Every client I've had who had a hip replacement admitted that his or

---

[80] "Sitting At Your Desk Is Killing You. Here's What It Costs to Stop the Destruc-tion | Money.com." Accessed December 8, 2014.
http://time.com/money/2970619/sitting-at-your-desk-is-killing-you-heres-what-it-costs-to-stop-the-destruction/.

her pelvis was tight for decades. There is no drug that will release the tension that distorts your structure.

How to Reverse Structural Aging

Virtually all structural issues start as soft tissue contraction and restriction. Scoliosis, the lateral curvature of the spine, occurs from the muscles and fascia contracting unevenly.[81] Most structural aging comes from the stress of life or improper movement or posture. What our mothers, gym teachers, and drill sergeants taught us was wrong. "Standing up straight" creates an artificial appearance of good posture. Over time, it creates more tension and misalignment. For example, holding your "shoulders back" tightens your upper back and shoulders while making your head protrude forward.

Non-posture muscles aren't meant to HOLD you up – they are meant to move you quickly and easily in any direction. A contracted muscle restricts full movement. You may look like a good statue, standing erect, but you would be dead meat if a predator were stalking you.

Movement is the elixir of life. The Chinese stay young by doing Tai Chi (a simple movement exercise/martial art) in the park every day. They understand if you want to look and feel young, you need to move and release the tension in your body. The East Indians have their yoga. In the US, we have 90-year-old farmers who are out working their farms every day.

As good as it might feel and be for you, you don't need to go to a yoga class to bring movement back into your life. Start moving in irregular ways. Move sideways, backwards, on irregular surfaces at varied speeds. Get outside and hike a trail. For every 20 minutes of sitting, move for one minute.

---

[81] "Soft Tissue Release on the Concave Side in the Treatment of Scoliosis... - PubMed - NCBI." Accessed December 8, 2014. http://www.ncbi.nlm.nih.gov/pubmed/1597080.

The first movement you did is your most important: breathing. In more than three decades of treating patients, including Olympic runners, I never saw anyone who breathed to his or her full capacity. Focus on breathing in a relaxed manner. I don't mean breathe deeply, I mean breathe so that your entire upper body is relaxed, so you breathe a full breathe in and out. If there's one movement that can keep you young, it's the breath.

Start noticing where and when you hold your breath. Then relax. I guarantee the tension will come back, but over time of practicing relaxing and releasing, you will become more relaxed. From there your body will begin realigning and moving with more grace. You can cheat as I do, by getting others to help relax your body; try yoga, cranial-sacral therapy, massage, acupuncture, or Rolfing® SI.

Equipoise, a balance structure, is not necessarily a perfectly straight structure.[82] It's a body that is relatively aligned with gravity and moves with ease. I have clients who are in their 90s who are structurally young... so there is hope for you.

So What Is – Myofascial Release?

In the 1940s, a few obscure, forward-thinking osteopaths were working with fascia after it was first discovered that fascial adhesions were the cause of many conditions. But Dr. Ida P. Rolf made fascia famous. Dr. Rolf's new therapy, now known as Rolfing® SI, expanded what osteopaths understood about fascia, and what they could do to treat it.

Fascia is the thin, tough connective tissue that extends throughout the body from head to toe as a continuous three-dimensional web. Physical trauma, poor posture, prolonged stress, or inflammation force the fascia to bind up, twist, and constrict, creating scar tissue and leaving you

---

[82] For more on Structural Aging check out:
http://www.liberatedbody.com/valerie-berg-lbp-012/

with adhesions in your fascial system. These adhesions cause constriction around nerves, muscles, bones, blood vessels, and organs. That tightening pulls your body out of alignment, causing everything from back pain and poor, inefficient breathing to ankle and knee problems.

Traditional tests such as x-rays, myelograms, CAT scans, and electromyography don't show these restrictions. Because medical tests can't show fascial restrictions and their consequences, many people go undiagnosed. MRI's do produce images of soft tissue, but as friends of mine who are docs tell me—they don't often see what a Rolfer™ sees or feels. You should get these tests if there is a need, yet realize soft tissue even for Rolfers™ can be elusive.

Traditional medicine diagnoses and then treats symptoms—sore back, "bad" knee, whatever it is; Dr. Rolf, however, recognized the importance of focusing not on the symptoms, but on the fascial adhesions and their structural consequences.

Dr. Rolf also understood that you can't force change; the restriction will just return. Inevitably though, some practitioners thought that if a little pressure was good, then surely more would be better. The "old school" became associated with pain. Gentle Rolfing® SI evolved as the antithesis—more light massage or myofascial release than standard Rolfing® SI. Over the last decade, myofascial release has become popular. Practitioners claim that light pressure releases the adhesions.

There is a place for the more gentle approach. If you were working on a young child or the elderly, you would certainly be lighter. For the majority of clients, though, more pressure is often needed. The hallmark of effective Rolfing® SI is the slow, precise, and indirect pressure (following the tissue-releasing pattern) that sometimes may be firm. This combination of Dr. Rolf's firm approach, the sensitivity of osteopathic manipulation, the indirect manipulation of myofascial release, and cranio-sacral work creates the most powerful results.

In the beginning with any client, there will be a place or two that will need deep and precise pressure to get the tissue to release. Without genuine pressure, soft tissue that feels like bone will not release. It doesn't matter how much intent, time, or skill you apply. That hard, dead tissue needs pressure. I often see clients who have had work from a practitioner who used gentle pressure on these tougher areas. Other parts of the client might have changed, but these areas didn't.

I will do the more gentle manipulation when needed. I will also refer clients to cranial osteopaths, cranio-sacral therapists, and myofascial release practitioners when needed. That said, there is still a need to do deeper work on many people. My old friend, Denis Leri, is one of the original Feldenkrais practitioners. He's told me that Dr. Feldenkrais, the originator of this very gentle movement therapy, would, when needed, get in there to break up hard restrictions.

We learned that integrating the firmer pressure with slow indirect manipulation could be the most effective approach.

My caution—don't be lured into thinking gentle manipulation will do it all. When, as a Certified Rolfer™, you need to get the tissue released, go slow and go deep as you respond to the tissue releasing. As a client, trust a Certified Rolfer™ with the skill to go deep in an indirect manner. It can feel good, and it is certainly safe and effective.

Rolfing® SI Releases Chronic Stress

Nobel Prize winner Roger Sperry, Ph.D. nails it with this statement: "The most critical clinical effect of manipulative therapy[83] is the quieting of sympathetic hyperactivity."[84]

"Sympathetic hyperactivity" is when the "fight-or-flight" response kicks in when you're not in physical danger. Getting very stressed out over traffic when there is nothing life-threatening about being stuck in bumper-to-bumper traffic is one example.

---

[83] http://en.wikipedia.org/wiki/Manual_therapy

[84] http://en.wikipedia.org/wiki/Hyperactivity

So when the soft tissue relaxes, it releases the stored tension of the stress response and stops compressing the muscles and organs of the body. That compression restricts movement and circulation.

"I used to have horrible indigestion whenever I was tired," one of my clients told me. "Finally, one day, I realized that when I'm tired, I don't always sit or stand up straight. My stomach wasn't physically working right. Now when I have an upset stomach, the first thing I try is sitting up straight and breathing deeply. It usually works." His awareness, coupled with the release of his chronic tension, allowed him to change a chronic problem.

As the stored stress releases, the resources that went into being "hyperactive" can be allocated to rejuvenation. If your body is fighting the fight, it doesn't have those resources for your immune system.

Why are some people always sick? Why does it take others so long to get well? Why are so many people feeling old before their time? It is the structural and fascial restrictions that build up over the years perpetuating the chronic stress as a default state of existence.

The Good News

Through skillful manipulation of the soft tissue, this tension can be released. Rehab and exercise will not release *this* tension. Rolfing® SI can release the tension. The more chronic tension that is released, the quicker you get well. If the therapist is working on realigning your structure, you have the added benefit of not fighting the effects of gravity.

Anger – Is It Your Friend?

When was the last time you lost it? When you just said it like it is? A *New York Times* article, "The Benefits of Blowing Your Top[85]," reported on new research: apparently, expressing yourself can be good for you.

I lost it the other night. I can't say it felt good at the time. Part of me thought I should keep my mouth shut. But there was that other part of me that needed to speak, and I made a conscious choice to let that part have its say. As I was speaking, I wanted to explode. But I didn't. I simply explained to the person yelling at me, point by point, why his information was wrong. When I was done, I felt good.

After the man left, the other people at the meeting said, "I wish I'd said what you said." We then discussed how difficult it can be to articulate angry feelings. I know. For the first part of my life I perfected the art of shutting up. If I thought anyone else was going to get angry, I would move to the back of the room. I cowered in any confrontation. But 30 years ago, I finally got fed up with being a wimp. I remember how difficult speaking your feelings can be, and now I know how liberating speaking your feelings can be.

For 35 years, I have witnessed the price these repressed emotions have on our health and emotional wellbeing. The big things don't kill us; it's all of the accumulated little emotions we stuff down. I have good, resourceful people come to me so tense that they are ready to explode. Their blood pressure is off the charts, their backs and/or necks are killing them, and their GI tracks are rebelling against the stress by shutting down. Repressed emotions become stress, stress becomes tension, tension becomes tightness, and tightness becomes the thick fascia, which compresses joints and organs.

You are walking around in a body shrink-wrapped with emotional stress. When it is socially appropriate to express it, you can't. Your body and

---

[85] https://www.nytimes.com/2010/07/06/health/06mind.html

your emotions are conditioned to restrain rather than express. More stress builds, more tension is created to hold that stress in—you are doomed. Turn this around by noticing what you are doing or not doing. Breathe. Then at the risk of doing it wrong, start speaking. Usually the first few times it's a little rough. You will get better at it and it will get easier. No one will die. In fact, the truth might get out. Wouldn't that be liberating?

Are You Using Stress to Make You Strong?

When I owned a health care clinic in Phoenix, one of the things we offered was courses in Mindfulness Based Stress Reduction. We got the super Type-A executives and professionals referred by their doctors who were unsuccessful at helping them. Their blood pressure or anti-anxiety drugs might as well have been placebos. Stress was more than decreasing their quality of life; it was killing them.

After forty years of seeing the ravages of stress on my clients' lives, I do see that certain stressors serve us. Exercise is the best example of how stress makes us strong. Without movement that strains us, we become weak. Our muscles will atrophy, and our bones will disintegrate. Without the stress of learning, our mental abilities decrease.

Nassim Taleb's book Anti-Fragile[86] explains how discomfort allows you to bounce back stronger and elevate your performance. *Hormesis* is the biological phenomenon what allows you to improve your health and grow from exposure to minor doses of an agent that is otherwise toxic or lethal when given at higher doses. Sunlight and its gamma-rays and UV-radiation is good in low dosage; we need sunlight to synthesize Vitamin D. But we all know what can happen when we get too much sun.

---

[86] http://amzn.com/1400067820

How to Benefit from Hormesis

As the basis for all athletic and psychological improvement, hormesis can be the catalyst that breaks you out of a plateau of mediocrity. Your homeostasis can gradually degrade into death if your body or mind is not challenged. For instance, without the stress of gravity, an astronaut's bones disintegrate.

The negative effects of stress come from the input that the body can't grow or learn from. It might not be the intensity of the stress, but its duration that causes disease. So, how do you know if the stress you are experiencing is good for you?

If your body is not going into prolonged stress response—that is, a survival response of fight, flight, or freeze—then you aren't accumulating stress. If your body/mind is using the stress to develop new behaviors, whether cellular or global, then hormesis is at play. Simply, if you can't leverage stress to develop a new behavior that enhances your life, end the stressful behavior.

One of the key components of hormesis is how it produces a release of tension or toxins. Rolfing clients will often come to see me because they are in chronic pain that no drug or treatment will relieve. Maybe their back pain reached a point where walking is a major feat. What surprises these clients is how tight and sensitive their backs are to my touch. A light touch might produce a jerk. Slowly over a few sessions, what was highly sensitive is now relaxing.

Using the stimulus of my touch to trigger a release not only made their body less sensitive, but released the tension causing their chronic back pain. Allowing for the pain in the beginning of the treatments caused the tension to release. In the process of releasing the chronic tension, these clients learned how to prevent new stress from producing new tension. None of this would be possible without allowing what was negative to be the healing agent. What in your life that is a negative can you use to enhance it? How can you vary your lifestyle to encourage your body to be more resilient?

Owen Marcus

Rolfing's® SI Connection to Dermatitis

As a Certified Rolfer™, clients don't generally come to me because of dermatitis, but over the years some of my clients have had it. And I've learned something interesting: often the cause of chronic dermatitis is beneath the skin.

Contact dermatitis occurs after exposure to an external irritant. Most *chronic* dermatitis, however, is caused by something the body is producing. In response to stress or through the body's attempt to detoxify itself through the skin, the body creates and releases a toxic substance that irritates the skin from the inside.

Occasionally, during a series of Rolfing® SI sessions, a client will go through a short period of having pimples or a little rash as the body releases whatever toxins were stored in the tissue. For years, studies have shown the body stores toxins such as DDT in its tissue. When circulation is returned to an area that was tense, the blood flushes out what was stored there. If our primary detoxifying organs—the liver, kidneys, and spleen—can't handle the load, other organs such as the lungs, large intestine, and skin try to help.

You may not even realize that your body produces its own toxins. Even that natural survival response (stress), produces its own potentially toxic chemicals. With minor stress continuing over time, the body tenses and accumulates the byproducts of stress. Ever heard of a "stress rash?" Now you know what causes it; the skin is trying to release the stress-produced toxins that the other organs can't handle.

As an emotional organ, the skin reflects our stress and emotional state. We live in such a stress-filled culture; it's no surprise that 30 million Americans experience dermatitis every year.

Eliminating chronic dermatitis usually means detoxifying the body through herbs, bodywork, sweating, and nutrition. By strengthening the primary detoxifying organs and the body's general level of health, the burden is off the skin. Teaching our bodies how to better deal with stress is always important. And, as always, breathing always helps.

Skin problems are not usually life threatening, but if you suffer from dermatitis, you want to get well. Many years ago, a top dermatologist in Arizona was one of my clients. We repeatedly spoke about how stress was a huge cause of skin problems. He really cared about his patients, and he was often frustrated to find that he could not fully *heal* them because he couldn't reduce their stress levels.

Turning Insomnia Around

Each of us at some point in our life has experienced a night where we just could not seem to fall asleep. Whether from excitement, worry, or too much caffeine, we know the drain a lack of a good night's sleep can have on our energy level, as well as on our mental and emotional state. Imagine experiencing that on a regular basis. Based on 2007 figures from the US Department of Health and Human Services, approximately 64 million Americans suffer from insomnia on a regular basis each year—and it is 1.4 times more common in women than men.

The Problem

By definition, insomnia is a symptom of a sleeping disorder characterized by persistent difficulty falling asleep or staying asleep even though one has the opportunity to do so. It typically results in the individual experiencing some form of functional impairment while awake. Insomnia sufferers may also complain of an inability to close their eyes or "rest their mind" for more than a few minutes at a time. There are various types of insomnia. They include the following:

- *Transient* – may last from a few days to weeks and may result from changes in environment (i.e. time zone), schedule, depression, or stress.

- *Acute* – characterized by inability to sleep well for a period of three weeks to six months.

- *Chronic* – characterized with inability to sleep consistently for over a year's time.

In any of these situations, insomnia may be the primary concern or it may be a symptom of another disorder of a physiological or mental/emotional nature. There are a variety of possible causes for insomnia. As stated earlier, stress in the form of anxiety, depression, or even excitement can be a significant factor. Caffeine intake can also contribute to insomnia. Chronic pain can also contribute to disturbed sleep. This is widely reported in patients suffering from fibromyalgia, for example. Insomnia can also be associated with various hormonal imbalances affecting the thyroid, the adrenal glands, estrogen levels, or combinations thereof. Neurological disorders may also present with sleep disturbances, as can certain digestive and intestinal conditions.

Because insomnia is associated with so many different conditions, it is a good idea to first try to identify the underlying cause or contributing factors when seeking treatment.

A Solution

When was the last time you had a good night's sleep? If you're like the 64 million Americans suffering from insomnia on a regular basis, it might have been awhile. I've had clients come to me for help alleviating their insomnia. Fortunately for them, they realized that in order to treat chronic insomnia, they first had to tackle the primary cause: stress.

Other causes of insomnia include: too much caffeine; drugs (such as long-term sleep medication); hormonal imbalances; parasites; eating late at night. If you spend day after day wound up and stressed out, lying in bed might not be enough to slow you down.

I have observed clinically that what some people think of as relaxation is actually exhaustion. When you push yourself beyond your limit, your adrenals kick in to produce adrenalin and cortisol, leaving you so wired that you can't turn off your brain or body at night.

Exercise can help insomnia—if you're not doing it while exhausted! When I was in Scottsdale, I treated a lot of exhausted runners. Their pattern was: wake up exhausted, run to get going, push all day, come home exhausted but wired, and sleep poorly. Needless to say, they weren't healthy or well-rested.

When you're continually stressed, your stress chemicals never leave your system. The hormones are at such high levels and the organs that neutralize them are so burned out, the chemicals stay in your blood even when you don't need them. Additionally, the constant stress makes you so tense that even when the stress is gone, your body remains tight.

If you're stressed during the day, you need to de-stress before bed. Light yoga, a hot bath, or a massage from your partner can help relax you, and thereby help break the cycle of insomnia.

New habits = better sleep. If you really want to overcome insomnia, you have to be willing to change your habits. Years ago, a client came to me because getting to sleep was difficult for him, and when he did finally fall asleep, it wasn't restful. One of my first questions to him was "When do you eat dinner?" He told me that it was generally after 9 pm. I asked him why so late; he said that was the only time he was hungry. I explained to him that waking up not hungry was due to eating late, and he was only hungry at night because he was rushing around all day. I told him that without changing his eating habits, no treatment was going to help him sleep. I said I would not continue to see him until he changed. He never came back.

How do you break your cycle? Change the behaviors that are keeping you from sleeping. Eat early in the evening. Get exercise when you're rested. Cut back on caffeine. Take time to really relax before you go to bed. And learn to breathe.

Proper Breathing Is a Short-Cut

The simplest behavior change is learning to breath. Breathing naturally prevents stress from accumulating and releases chronic stress. None of the clients or students I've seen—including Olympic runners!—were breathing at their full capacity.

A deep, natural breath should result in movement of the front, side, and back of your abdomen and chest. Learning to relax so you can breathe this natural breath is one of the major benefits of Rolfing® SI or other good bodywork. Most of my clients come back after their first session and tell me they are sleeping better than they have in years. Bottom-line: When the body relaxes, the mind relaxes. When you're relaxed, sleep is easy.

How to Buy the Right Bed

Humans are designed to sleep on our backs, on hard ground. But we sleep on our sides or stomachs because of either a bad back or a bad bed. Healing that bad back is not the focus of this chapter, though; so what makes a good bed?

Well, bad beds are soft beds. A soft bed is like a hammock that sags. A night on your back in a sagging bed will surely produce an aching back in the morning.

A firm bed mimics sleeping on the ground, but lying flat is uncomfortable for people who have tight backs. People with bad backs want a softer bed so they aren't crushing their shoulders when they sleep on their sides; a softer bed allows the pelvis to drop down into the bed more allowing the spine to be straighter while on your side. This is the picture you often see in bed ads touting their special bed—but it's actually not good for you.

Assuming you want a bed that will encourage you to sleep on your back, I recommend latex. I have a latex mattress I purchased more than 25 years ago and it's still firm. Latex is natural rubber[87] and it doesn't off-gas like foam; it's also antimicrobial. It breathes and it lasts.

---

[87] http://en.wikipedia.org/wiki/Natural_rubber

Also, you don't need box springs. That's a bunch of marketing hype. Don't blame the mattress sales people though—they're trained to tell you that. They probably really believe that buying a mattress without a box spring will ruin "your investment." But my bed is a platform bed[88], just a mattress, no box spring, and it is 25 years old.

Some people like futons[89] because they are cheap and versatile. But the standard cotton futons get very hard very fast as they compact. Since the mattress lies on planks, not a platform, you get some spots that are harder than others and it can feel like you're lying on steel bars.

Memory foam[90] is popular, too, but it releases a lot of gases and can be hot to sleep on because it doesn't breathe at all.

Bottom line: you need to test drive your mattress. Lying on it for a couple minutes in a store doesn't work. If you're spending hundreds—or even thousands—of dollars on a mattress, get a guarantee that you can return it after a month if you don't like it. You only have one back. You can buy another mattress.

Pelvic Floor Problems

Most would associate pelvic floor problems with urinary incontinence, but actually they are your sex muscles. It is difficult to have good sex without good pelvic floor tone. By tone I am not speaking of strength in the sense of hard and tight. I am speaking about soft tissue being like the muscles of a cat, relaxed and strong.

Susan Gala, the developer of **Sex*her*cise – Feminine Fitness from Within**™ understands how to get un-toned pelvic floor[91] muscles back in shape. Check out her site and blog at www.pelvicfloorexercise.net.

---

[88] http://en.wikipedia.org/wiki/Platform_bed

[89] http://en.wikipedia.org/wiki/Futon

[90] http://en.wikipedia.org/wiki/Memory_foam

I met Susan at a book writing conference in N.Y.C. She impressed me with her understanding of the pelvic floor and how to tone it. As a Certified Rolfer™ I know what Susan says is true:

> As females we may be at risk of developing pelvic floor problems, such as stress, incontinence, pelvic floor weakness, or pain during intimacy. Life events such as childbirth, menopause, poor diet, or the natural aging process can cause changes in our pelvic floor muscles. Stronger pelvic floor muscles can improve stress incontinence, a condition affecting over 12 million women in the US.

Rolfing® SI is not the only way to release and tone your pelvic floor. It might be one of the quickest ways, but there are many other programs from exercise to visceral manipulation. I've seen women and men well into their 60's experiencing the best sex of their lives in part because their pelvic floors had the proper tone. Both men's and women's hyper-tonicity and hypo-tonicity of the pelvic floor is dependent on the rest of the pelvic structure and related areas. Tension in the pelvis, hips, legs, and abdomen will affect the pelvic floor. All of these structures may be tight or some may be tight and restrictive, while others may be loose and hyper-mobile (see How to Heal Your Old Sprains and Strains). As Rolfers™ we don't directly work on the pelvic floor, but releasing and organizing these other structures often results in pelvic floor changes.

How to Get Flexible

Are you flexible? I certainly wasn't 35 years ago—before I tried Rolfing® SI. I couldn't cross my legs while sitting in a chair, my walk was a waddle, and my body's soft tissue felt more like a cedar tree.

Baby-boomers annually suffer from more than 1 million sports injuries which cost over $20 billion dollars in medical expenses each year. We

---

[91] http://en.wikipedia.org/wiki/Pelvic_floor

can assume that many of those injuries could have been prevented or reduced if these people were more flexible.

How to Get Flexible – Way One

There are essentially two ways—do it yourself or hire some to do it for you. The first step is stretching—great way to keep flexible. Getting a 30-year-old, tight body to become loose through stretching can be slow at best, but it can happen if the person goes slowly and consistently and gets coaching from someone who knows what she's doing.

All too often a fellow will do a few stretches only to injure himself. What he didn't realize was that once the fascia becomes scar tissue, it will not release when stretched. If anything releases, it is the place of least resistance, which may be too hyper-mobile to start with. This is most prevalent with knees. I have seen hundreds of runners, cyclists, and other athletes come in with chronic knee problems, many after surgeries, physical therapy, and personal training. Their knees continued to get looser and looser as the rest of them became tighter.

Don't get me wrong… all of these treatments are valid disciplines providing needed help. Unfortunately, they don't release the chronic soft tissue tension built up over years of stress and repetitive motion.

Slow, precise, and consistent stretching can help the body begin to release this tension. Having someone who is trained in a method that focuses on releasing through relaxation can achieve this goal. Most of us guys are not strong on patience, but that is starting to change. I am seeing more and more men get into yoga. These men aren't looking for the quick fix. They understand if they are to get benefits from yoga, they need to have good instruction and stick to it.

How to Get Flexible – Way Two

The second method—hiring someone to do it for you—is faster. Body-work such as massage, Feldenkrais[92], and Rolfing® SI are the three most common therapies to transform a tight body into a loose one. Compared to stretching, these therapies are more passive and focus on the critical areas. And I lied a bit—there is some work on your part with these therapies. At the very least, you have to get yourself to their office.

In my experience, the area that is in pain is virtually never the primary site of a chronic injury. Usually that pain area needs some work, but if the work is to be sustained, other areas need to be addressed. Good bodywork will take this systemic approach and not just keep treating the symptom.

I have seen ex-professional football players, some of the tightest athletes I have ever treated, end up with a loose and flexible body that they had previously thought impossible to achieve. As long as the problem is in the soft tissue, it can change. Some tight bodies just take longer.

How to Cheat at Yoga

The growing popularity of yoga, with more than 11 million Americans doing yoga regularly, has Americans doing what we do best—improving efficiency through innovation.

In a matter of two decades, yoga has become 'the new running' not only for aging baby boomers, but also for our younger generations. Because of our rush to excel, we enhance, heat up, or just intensify traditional yoga. As we transform yoga into more of a sport, we also realize that our western bodies don't perform poses like we think we should.

---

[92] http://en.wikipedia.org/wiki/Feldenkrais_Method

Think about it: yoga comes from a culture where people often sit on the floor and start their yoga practice as young children. When you take a 40-year-old man that has stretched a total of an hour his whole life, a little difficulty is to be expected. So, what's a typical first response when resistance is met? That's right, we do it harder, especially us men. And what happens when new yogis can't release and relax by straining more? Many quit.

Ways to Cheat

Some people are discovering remedial ways to take tight western bodies and loosen them, so what might take 10 years of yoga can occur in less than one. They do this by releasing the soft tissue[93] restrictions through therapies that specifically release chronic tension. This can make a significant difference in how a body benefits from yoga. When you can take a hamstring that feels like a steel cable and turn it into to a soft bungee cord, you improve your ability to effectively practice yoga.

By releasing chronic tension through precise pressure, the body slowly relaxes that tension in a way yoga can't for a tight body. For a chronically tight body, stretching the tightness will have limited effects. Yet, once that body starts to relax, what was once torture in yoga becomes pleasure.

Over 25 years ago I had a judge come to me for Rolfing® because his wife's yoga class showed him that despite his running success, he had a body of stone. Because he immediately saw improvements with Rolfing®, he was a good student. He learned to completely change his running stride so he actually became looser from running. After ten Rolfing® sessions and a year of integrating the sessions, he went back to yoga. Immediately, he was one of the loosest men in the class.

---

[93] http://en.wikipedia.org/wiki/Soft_tissue

Cheating (by releasing tension) can:

- Turn hard tissue soft

- Prevent hyper-mobilization and cheating during yoga poses

- Teach your body to relax

- Allow you to relax

- Allow you to get into new yoga positions

- Prevent injuries

- Quicken and enhance the benefits of yoga

- Release and then allow you to strengthen your core muscles without tightening

A body that is virtually never stretched can't be expected to perform like the body of someone who has been doing yoga for 20 years. Don't make it hard on yourself—get help! I love yoga. I recommend it to most of my clients. In addition to being a great way to stay loose, it will keep you fit and young. You might need a little help to prime your yoga pump, but even the yoga instructors I've Rolfed over the years will swear to the benefits of releasing the chronic tension and the resulting improvements to their yoga.

Do You Know the Secret to Boosting Your Immune System?

Posture Is the Key
When we talk about "immune boosters," an important one usually gets left out: good posture. Having good structure and healthy connective tissue helps keep you well. How efficiently your body is organized and in alignment with gravity directly impacts your health and immune system:

Better than 90% of the energy output of the brain is used in relating the physical body to/within its gravitational field. The more mechanically distorted a person is, the less energy is available for thinking, metabolism, and healing [the immune system].

-Dr. Roger Sperry, 1980 Nobel Prize for Brain Research

You may not realize how much effort you are exerting to "hold yourself up" and move. You gradually accumulate stress and tension. It builds so slowly that you don't consciously experience its full impact. Plus, everyone around us is doing the same thing, so your experience of "getting old" seems normal. But the resources that are diverted to standing and walking incorrectly can deplete immune resources.

How Is Your Kid's Posture?

Who told you to stand up straight? Was it your mom? Was it your gym teacher or drill sergeant? Did you listen? Hopefully, you didn't.

Over the years in seeing more than a thousand Rolfing® SI clients, I have never had one person come in standing straight despite the nagging.

The truth is the cues you were given—hold your shoulders back, suck your stomach in, push your chest out, tuck your pelvis under—those are all stress responses. Even if you're not stressed, if you're standing in that posture, you became stressed. You aren't breathing naturally; your breath is restricted by holding your pelvis, stomach, and shoulders unnaturally.

When you maintain a posture behavior long enough, it becomes unconscious and eventually a fixed structure. The fact that everyone around you is doing some version of the same thing is not helping. On top of this, posture can be a form of expression. We see this particularly with teenagers. Often their slouching is a form of defiance, an indirect assertion of their independence. Our requests to, "Stand up straight!" are futile.

For kids, when they add carrying heavy backpacks (particularly on one shoulder), wearing flip flops, bad ergonomics, and reading lying down, they are increasing the likelihood of back and neck problems. Slouching, which kids are masters at, will add to these problems.

If these weren't bad enough, let me add another variable: you. We all learn posture from our parents. You might have been told that your big thighs were inherited from your dad and your flat feet from your mom. That was what I was told. I believed it until I saw a Certified Rolfer™ and saw my legs magically drop 20 pounds of tension and my feet develop an arch. I realized I didn't inherit these characteristics, I learned them. I *developed* the walk of my father, which gave me his tight legs.

Years ago I had a client, David, with a bad groin problem that was easy to fix with Rolfing® SI. About a year later, David asked if I could help his son. It turned out his son had the same structure and movement pattern David had when he first came in. His son never had the injury David had, he just modeled his father and ended up with the same groin pain!

How to Achieve Better Posture

Correcting bad posture by unnaturally holding your body tighter *might* have you or your child standing straighter, but all of you will end up more tensed. My first step with clients is to point out the things they're doing that are adding to their problem. Their self-corrections will shift one area only to put some other area further out of whack.

Next I show them with their own body how to stand relaxed. Everyone is leaning back without realizing it. Of course it doesn't feel that way or you would shift it. In fact, when I put you straight you'll feel like you're leaning forward—but a mirror or photo will show you that you're actually straight. That little shift can make the difference for some clients.

Once you are "forward," you can begin to relax your stomach. This is much harder for adults than kids. Not only have we been told to hold it in, we want to hold it in to look good. We create a girdle of tension. (As an aside, not only are girdles for women coming back, but now there are girdles for men. We put aesthetics before health.)

Next I have my clients relax their shoulders. Many of us hold them up around our ears. Those neck and upper back muscles were not meant to constantly hold your shoulders and arms up. The shoulder girdle is meant to sit on the rib cage. Most people hold their shoulders back, which increases upper back tension and makes for even more shallow breathing.

Most people's necks are tilted forward unnaturally. But pulling your neck back will only produce more tension because your neck is forward to compensate for the fact that your chest is back as a result of the whole body being tilted back and also often from slouching. When your chest is stacked above the pelvis, your neck can naturally readjust to the correct position above the chest.

You or your child can get help from a yoga instructor, Feldenkrais practitioner, or a Certified Rolfer™ to assist in creating better posture. Learning the *Natural Walk* (see section later in book) is the quickest way to teach yourself to have better posture. Play with the walk. Watch others walk and stand. See how many times in a day you can self-correct. If you were fully relaxed, you would be perfectly straight... without effort.

How Is Your Inflammation Killing You?

Research continues to point to inflammation as a cause or strong co-cause for most illnesses. It is not the acute inflammation of an injury that is a concern, but rather chronic inflammation[94] that produces diseases such as obesity, diabetes, dementia[95], depression and cancer. A recent study showed that elderly subjects who had the highest levels of C-reactive protein and interleukin 6 (two markers of systemic inflammation) were 260% more likely to die in four years.

---

[94] http://en.wikipedia.org/wiki/Inflammation

[95] http://www.ultrawellness.com/blog/9-steps-to-reverse-dementia

You can continue to treat the effects of inflammation—or you can treat the cause. The cause is an irritant, which is a stressor to the body. It might be a repetitive motion injury, an allergen, a toxin or the psychological stress of life.

Along with inflammation, the body produces scar tissue, be it in the blood vessel or the fascia of your leg. You see it in that bad ankle sprain you had many years ago. First, it hurt like hell and swelled up. Today you are left with a thicker retinaculum, a band of fascia around the tendons above the ankle. Over time, full range of motion is restricted while making your ankle more vulnerable to strains.

Mark Hyman, MD wrote an excellent article[96] explaining the role of inflammation in disease and what you can do to not only prevent disease, but also stay young. He doesn't address what Rolfing® SI addresses, the soft tissue system. Your connective tissue is as vulnerable to inflammation as your blood vessels and colon. If your C-reactive protein (the measure for inflammation) levels are high not only are you at risk of cardiovascular disease and death, you are more likely to have joint and soft tissue pain because of chronic inflammation.

After watching his video or reading his posts, you will better understand how chronic irritation produces chronic inflammation which leads to disease and, according to Hyman, "rapid aging." He gives 7 Steps to Living an Anti-inflammatory Life:

1. Whole Foods

2. Healthy Fats

3. Regular Exercise

---

[96] http://drhyman.com/blog/2010/06/01/is-your-body-burning-up-with-hidden-inflammation/

4. Relax

5. Avoid Allergens

6. Heal Your Gut

7. Supplement

As Certified Rolfers™, we help release the stressors of misalignment, movement maladaptation, and the emotional stress stored in the soft tissue recreating more stress. A body which has experienced Rolfing® SI not only contains less stress, it is also more adaptable to stress, thereby being less "irritated." Without constant irritation, there is no inflammation and scarring.

As Hyman says, deal with the cause. Don't keep treating the symptoms with a litany of drugs.

Arthritis

Each of us has friends and family that say they suffer from arthritis. It is so common today that we take it for granted. With the maturing of the "boomers" we have begun to expect arthritis as part of the aging experience.

Research is uncovering that arthritis now affects people as early as age 25. One of the professional dental assistants I have recently been visiting shared with me that her three-year old daughter is suffering from juvenile rheumatoid arthritis. I was stunned to hear that.

Arthritis is generally considered an inflammation of the joints leading to pain or tenderness, stiffness, perhaps localized swelling, sometimes a crunchiness sound in the joints known as crepitus. There is often a loss of full range of motion in the affected areas: the neck, shoulders, elbows, wrists, hands, hips, knees, and ankles. This occurs because joint spaces become narrowed due to a loss of cartilage or crystalline boney deposits. Wear and tear, normal for active people, as well as repetitive motions experienced in work and sports activities, accumulates as we age and may cause damage to the collagen matrix covering and padding our joint ends.

The bone, cartilage, tendons, ligaments, fluids, etc. which comprise our joints are always moving to enable our actions. Stress and strain on our joints can cause damage that in turn causes irritation and thus inflammation. Surfaces that were once smooth become rough, irritated, and tender. Such inflammation alerts the body to release enzymes that further damage the irritated cartilage. Two forms of arthritis are more familiarly recognized: Osteoarthritis (OA) and Rheumatoid Arthritis (RA).

You might ask yourself, "If I am living a normal active lifestyle, what causes me to acquire such a condition?" Some causes may be a congenital predisposition, such as abnormalities in joint or bone structures, as arthritis tends to run in families. Also: trauma, obesity (whereby excess weight places additional wear on weight bearing joints), nutritional deficiencies, illness or disease (even previously experienced ones that leave an "imprint" on structures), allergies, immune disorders, stress (and who doesn't experience stress in our busy lives), and our everyday exposures to environmental pollutants and toxins.

Most of these "symptoms" are addressed with pain relieving medications, and many work well in spite of the variety of side effects. But the causes are the real culprits that must be addressed for long lasting relief.

Natural therapies have become more widespread in reducing the pain, swelling, stiffness, and loss of mobility in affected joints and can work in complement with ongoing medical interventions. Our exposures to industrial pollutants and toxins have led to many disorders affecting digestion, all with a connection to OA and RA, such as leaky gut syndrome, GERD (Gastroesophageal reflux disease), candidiasis (overgrowth of yeasts in the gut), allergies, chemical sensitivities, chronic infections, and autoimmune disorders such as AS (ankylosing spondylitis) and lupus erythematosis.

In my practice, I've worked with many people who were diagnosed with arthritis. After Rolfing® SI, the symptoms usually went away when the soft tissue tension left. In this country, we traditionally have little understanding of how soft tissue affects all aspects of our existence. A few years ago, my colleagues produced the first international conference on fascia[97] at Harvard Medical School for clinicians and researchers. Each subsequent conference explored more deeply the importance fascia has on our health.

Often, someone who has osteoarthritis will tell me that the joint they injured many years ago is now the joint with arthritis. Previous trauma creates a cascade of body responses that can end with a joint locking up. By releasing the effect of the trauma in the soft tissue, we can often prevent arthritis. In a small number of cases, this has led to reversing arthritis. I will be the first to admit, however, that after a joint has deteriorated, removing the soft tissue strain may be of little benefit to the joint. Yet Rolfing® SI can prevent other areas from tightening.

Natural Walking and Running – Structural Integration, The Journal of the Rolf Institute®

This article appeared in the June 2011 issue of Structural Integration, The Journal of the Rolf Institute®. *It offers a technical explanation of my Natural Walking and Running.*

Introduction

The first thing I teach all of my clients is how to breathe. When I can get my clients breathing correctly, it helps them manage their stress, and hopefully they won't need me anymore. After breathing, the next thing I work on is walking. Breathing is an instinctual behavior; walking is only partly instinctual, as much of it is modeled. We watch our parents walk, and we copy their movement style as well as the emotional style embodied in their movement. Some of us may rebel against our parents to create an opposing style (picture the rebellious, slouching teenager).

---

[97] http://fasciacongress.org/

Either way, we are in some manner being affected by how and why our parents walk a particular way.

In this culture we study walking and running biometrically, yet we still don't understand how to do either correctly. For whatever reason, we adopted a walking style that created a limited approach to dealing with gravity. To compensate, we created high-tech shoes that soften our walk and encourage us to walk and run incorrectly. Propelled by these shoe companies and our mechanistic paradigm of human movement, we created reductionist models of how humans are meant to move.

Why the Natural Walk™?

As Certified Rolfers™, we all tend to agree that this "civilized" model of walking is not working. It might be good for generating clients for our practice, but it's not good for human bodies. We've forgotten something so simple: how to walk and run like an indigenous person.

Possibly the most brilliant focus of Dr. Rolf's work was her emphasis on gravity. Just as fish are not aware of water, we are not aware of gravity—or at least we weren't before Rolf championed the importance of not just relating to gravity, but using it. Back in the 1970s when I was training to become a Certified Rolfer™, I had sessions in Rolf Movement™ (or, as it was called then, Patterning) with Megan James and Heather Heartsong (Wing). Both taught me how to let gravity work for me. I've practiced Rolfing® Structural Integration for more than thirty years with no injuries to myself—and I credit them. I also credit them with planting the seeds of "Natural Walking."

Soon after I opened my practice in Scottsdale, Arizona, in 1980, I started seeing runners as clients. Their injuries taught me what *not* using gravity can do to a body. Regardless of orthotics, new shoes, or knee surgeries, their injuries would return. And it wasn't just my clients: up to eight out of every ten runners are hurt *every year*.[98] Rolfing® SI and reorganizing their structures weren't enough. With Rolfing® SI they improved more and they went longer between injuries, but the injuries could still return.[99] I tried teaching Rolf Movement™, but I wasn't getting through to them. Maybe it was too theoretical, or maybe it was how I was teaching it. Regardless, I needed to come up with a way to build on the principles of Rolfing® SI and Rolf Movement™ that these runners would understand and practice.

Maybe it's my dyslexia, but I'm a simple man, so I look for simple solutions. One day as I was explaining these principles to a runner, I showed him how to just fall forward. In my exaggeration, he understood. He tried it a few times in my office. When he came back the next week, he was starting to embody the fall. Over the course of a few more sessions, he mastered falling forward. I knew I had something when he reported that he was running pain-free, faster, and enjoying it once again.

Why Now?

With the resurging interest in Rolfing® SI and the barefoot running craze, there is a new opportunity to step in and help runners in a simple way. Who better to speak about gravity, structure, and movement than a Certified Rolfer™?

I suspect you're also seeing clients more frustrated than ever before with the institutional answers they have been given for years. People are smart. When you explain to them how something works, they get it. When you tell them that we're not meant to fight gravity, we're meant to use it, they get it. People want easy, low-tech, and inexpensive ways to enjoy their bodies.

---

[98] McDougall gives a beautiful description of a Tarahumara Indian running his natural run.

[99] McDougall, op. cit., pg. 170. "Every year anywhere from 65-89% of all runners suffer an injury."

From a professional and marketing perspective, I found work with runners to be very rewarding. Yes, some can be neurotic about running. The upside is that they are all very aware of their performance, so when you improve their performance, they know it! Over the years, I have done running clinics teaching Natural Running to clients and non-clients. Everyone gets it. All of them apply it in some way.

As you start teaching Natural Running, you'll become a local expert and resource for the running community and beyond. My Phoenix practice took off once I started helping local runners. Until they receive this kind of help, runners' injuries will continue to get worse and worse. Eventually, some will have to stop running. The runners you help will become your best advertising, telling all their injured friends how you did more good than the six pairs of orthotics or the running coaches.

The Development of Natural Walking and Running

I will not go into the biomechanical theories or research behind Natural Walking or Running, as Certified Rolfers™ Gael Ohlgren and David Clark wrote a thorough article on the science behind Natural Walking.[100] I used my clients as my beta testers and began to see that the more I simplified what I told and showed them, the quicker they got it. I knew I was getting it when these clients were teaching their friends what they had learned from me.

After a few years of success with runners, Arizona State University's Exercise Physiology Department approached me about doing a study with elite runners. They randomly divided the participating men into three groups: a control group, who received no treatment; a group who received ten regular massages; and the group that received Rolfing® SI sessions.

---

[100] Ohlgren, Gael and David Clark, "A Certified Rolfer™'s Response to Gracovetsky." Structural Integration: The Journal of the Rolf Institute®, vol. 37, issue 4, Dec. 2009, pp. 31-37. Also available at http://rolfhub.com/2010/03/05/natural-walking/.

I warned the researchers that their measurements, such as shank angle (angle of the ankle), were just measurements of the parts and not the functioning of the whole body. They assured me that these biomechanical measurements would show any improvements there were. As it turned out, there were no significant differences in measurements between any of the groups, yet every runner in the Rolfing® SI group saw his injuries disappear and set new personal records. Unfortunately, the researchers were focused entirely on biomechanical indicators, and did not measure the injury reductions or the performance improvements.

Principles

It's All About Gravity.

Using gravity to move forward is a simple concept, but teaching it can be tricky. The part my clients find the most difficult is to surrender to gravity, letting go and falling forward. It's difficult to shift from decades of leaning back ("Stand up straight!" "Square those shoulders!") to leaning into life, trusting that if you lean forward, you won't fall. It's no different than a new skier learning to lean into the "fall-line," that imaginary line of gravity pulling him down the mountain. Every cell in your body is saying, "If I lean forward, I'll fall flat on my face."

I use Natural Walking as an opportunity to increase the ease of breathing and body-awareness clients have developed from Rolfing® SI. As they start to get the walk, I keep reminding them to breathe a full, relaxed breath. I want their walk to be a subtle meditation of breath and gravity. This is a great way to metaphorically set the person up for bigger surrenders and changes. Inevitably, as a client starts to get the walk down, he or she starts to lean more into life.

Core Movement

Now that every trainer is a "core strength trainer," we see clients come to us shortened and tightened from "strengthening their core." I use Natural Walking and running to teach clients what the core muscles are and how to use them for the ultimate core exercise. Sometimes, I tell them stories about Rolf's "psoas walk." When they relax and let gravity do the work, the body is positioned in such a way that the core muscles are used and the sleeve muscles are only secondary supporters on level ground. Walking and running correctly will make a person's core stronger without making it shorter or tighter.

Simple Concepts

A simple model allows the client to focus more on his body. These are the ways I communicate my key points:

Breath: A relaxed breath is required to fully embody this walk:

- A relaxed breath goes from the floor of the pelvis up the front, sides, and back of the trunk to the neck.

- Allow yourself to feel whatever is tense, and then relax it. Once you relax one area, you may feel another tense area. Relax it. This doesn't mean you are holding. It means either your old unconscious pattern returned and now you are aware of it, or that the next layer of chronic tension wants to release.

- Holding tension is a waste of energy that restricts the body, making it less efficient. By letting go, your body inevitably becomes more efficient.

- Breathe like a baby.

Use gravity: Let gravity do the work by pulling you forward.

- Feel how gravity wants you to move forward.

- Imagine you are a caveman man out for a walk. Forget all the other instructions others told you about how to walk. Go primitive.

- After breathing, learning to use gravity was the next behavior you started learning. Now you get to master it.

- To run, lean forward more, surrender more, and you'll go faster. Let your legs be spokes on a wheel.

- Allow your body to be erect and relaxed while leaning forward from your ankles.

- Don't work. Let gravity do it.

Find your sweet spot: Go to where you are in your zone of minimal effort and maximum results.

- Keep letting go with your breath, lean into gravity, and let it get easier and easier.

- Use the negative feedback of tension or pain to direct you to pleasure and ease; i.e., when it hurts, readjust. (I have a client who knows when she is forgetting to lean forward while running, because she starts to get a headache. She adjusts her stride, leans into it again, and her headache goes away.)

- The entire experience becomes a movement meditation, surrendering and surrendering more.

- When you have surrendered, that peak experience can show up. This is where that runner's high comes in.

Cues and Shoes

I tense every time I hear "experts" give postural and movement instructions like this (ostensibly about natural walking): "Pull your shoulders back slightly. Keep your body perpendicular to the ground and walk tall. If you walk in a confident manner, you will gain confidence. With each step, land on your heel. Flex your foot and allow it to roll from heel to toes."[101] Through the Rolfing® SI process, I make a point of correcting misconceptions around good posture and proper walking.

---

[101] Sravani, "The Natural Way to Walk." Alternative Therapies, March 29, 2010, http://www.drgranny.com/fitness/the-natural-way-to-walk/.

I have found that trying to teach the *Natural Walk* directly rarely worked and that practicing an exaggerated form of it is the best way to create a new default walking form. By going overboard, you quickly extinguish the old proprioceptive anchors of what alignment is and what the correct walk is. When I demonstrate the exaggerated version, clients' first comment is usually, "No way. I'm not doing that. I'll look like a dork." But then I contrast this to the "shoulders back" command quoted above, and show how this forces the head forward and trunk back, while restricting breathing even further. I show clients that when we walk while leaning back, there is a natural tendency to counterbalance by holding the shoulders.

Understanding that shoulder, upper back, and neck tension can come from their walk, and that they can release that tension just by moving correctly, clients are more receptive and less worried about looking stupid.

There's also much to consider about our choice of shoes. Up until the 1950s and 1960s, high school cross-country teams training barefoot was commonplace.[102] Heel-striking became popular when that's what runners were told to do—particularly with the introduction of high-tech shoes. But heel strike transmits all the force of impact directly up through the leg, hip, and lower back. Over time, the weak links in a person's structural chain start to break. (As Certified Rolfers™, we are just about the only practitioners who don't keep trying to repair the weak links; rather, we strengthen the whole chain while, more importantly, decreasing the stress on it.)

We continue to create shoes either for the aesthetics (e.g., high heels), or we attempt to develop shoes to fix problems stemming from our

---

[102] McDougall, op. cit.

stride.[103] But recent research shows that the more expensive the running shoe, the worse the runner's injuries.

Daniel Lieberman, Ph.D., professor of biological anthropology at Harvard University, has been studying the growing injury crisis in the developed world for some time and has come to a startling conclusion: "A lot of foot and knee injuries currently plaguing us are caused by people running with shoes that actually make our feet weak, cause us to overpronate (ankle rotation), and give us knee problems."[104]

As if the return of the Earth Shoe, with its negative heel, is not bad enough, now we are seeing the rocker sole shoes with rounded bottoms meant to make the walker roll through her stride. Obviously, they must work for some people in the short-term, and the promise of a tighter butt is a strong selling point. They certainly are not promoting a natural stride or the development of a person's soft tissue and structure. They are the antithesis of the Vibram Five Fingers[105] shoes, removing all instinctive muscular development.

Nevertheless, long-held beliefs about walking and running are being questioned now with the popularity of barefoot running and the book *Born to Run.*[106] (They're still missing the most important piece of the puzzle though: the secret is leaning into gravity.) Writing about his experience with Vibram Five Fingers, one of the barefoot runner's shoes, a popular blog author relates: "The way to walk, these new experts claim, is to shorten the stride, keep the hips over the feet as much as possible,

---

[103] McDougall, op. cit., 168-179. The author weaves in several studies, expert opinions, and stories to show how the better the shoe, the worse the injury.

[104] McDougall, Christopher, "The painful truth about trainers: Are expensive running shoes a waste of money?" Mail Online, Feb. 22, 2011, http://www.dailymail.co.uk/home/moslive/article-1170253/The-painful-truth-trainers-Are-expensive-running-shoes-waste-money.html

[105] See examples at http://www.vibramfivefingers.com/barefoot-sports

[106] McDougall, op. cit.

and to land on the ball of the foot with the heel striking second. This method uses the foot and lower leg as nature intended—natural shock absorbers to minimize impact."[107]

Metaphors

In teaching new concepts I always look for metaphors that people understand experientially. One I use for Natural Walking and Running is Nordic skiing. I explain that your stride will look much like the stride of a cross-country skier who is leaning forward, stretching his leg out behind him. The skier wouldn't get anywhere if he were leaning back.

Many years ago, while in Arizona, I had a golf instructor as a client. A fellow Vermonter, he told me he'd tried Nordic skiing, but could never get the hang of it. It was obvious why when you saw him walk. If he'd been leaning any further back, he would have fallen over. He struggled with the walk for several weeks. As his body released and realigned, it became easier. One day he came in to proudly show me that he finally had it down. The *Natural Walk* had helped him in other areas too. He told me that for the first time, he was able to practice what he was preaching to his golf students: he could now easily get over the ball and swing from his lower body.

With skiers, I tell them to walk like they ski. Lean into the fall line. I steal Moshe Feldenkrais's line "stand like you are going to jump" as the setup for taking the first step, which is not a step. I show the client that the first act is not a step that puts him back; it's falling forward, which puts you in front of the vertical axis. We all want to start the movement with a controlled stride by extending the leg forward, rather than a fall. When the leg is forward, the torso shifts back behind the centerline. With the leg forward, we are leaning back, being pulled back by gravity,

---

[107] Hozaku, "Natural Walking and a Vibram Five Fingers Experiment." *Hozaku: Random ruminations*" [weblog], July 1, 2009, http://hozaku.com/post/Natural-Walking-and-a-Vibram-Five-Fingers-Experiment.aspx

rather than leaning toward where we want to go and having gravity propel us forward.

I joke with clients that I am teaching them to regress back to their ancestors. Our developed world is finally taking an important step backward in our ability to walk and run: our ancestors and the few indigenous peoples left are the ones who know how to walk and run efficiently and correctly. Humans evolved to be runners as much as we evolved as thinkers, or tool-users with an opposing digit. It was our ability to outrun any animal with our endurance that allowed us to survive.[108] I tell my clients to run like a hunter chasing down a gazelle.

Putting It Into Practice

I never see a client get the *Natural Walk* or Run without practice. There are a few that get it down in a week with minimal practice. Most, particularly us men, take weeks of exaggerating the walk or the run. I tell my clients to go someplace where they won't be recognized so they don't have to worry about looking stupid. I also emphasize practicing on a flat surface; walking or running up or down hills is a different stride. Irregular surfaces will be a distraction at first.

Fall forward from the ankles:

- It's all in the setup. Get straight—not what you thought was straight, but the Rolfing® straight, where there is a sense of lift.

- Imagine there are two sheets of plywood, one in front of you, one behind you, both hinged where your ankles are. Start gently rocking where only that hinge moves. Only your ankles are moving as you stand tall.

---

[108] Parker-Pope, Tara, "The Human Body Is Built for Endurance." *The New York Times*, Oct. 26, 2009, http://www.nytimes.com/2009/10/27/health/27well.html?_r=4&ref=health.

- Surrender. Let gravity do the work. Let gravity pull you forward as you relax and breathe.

- Lean forward and let gravity pull your back up and straight. When you lean forward there is a natural tendency to move out of a collapsed state and into straightening and lengthening.

- Fall.

- Allow one leg to be like a pole when you pole vault. You pivot over that leg as you fall. The other leg remains behind you, not pushing off. Then that second leg becomes the pivoting leg as you continue to fall.

- When the natural stride kicks in there is no sense of pushing off with the back leg on level ground. That leg pushes to pick up speed or to climb a hill. On level ground you feel very little effort coming from the rear leg. It is more like a rudder guiding the forward movement. The hind leg first starts bending not in the knee, but in the toes, foot, and ankle. The knee only bends once the weight is off the leg at the end of the stride for the rear leg.[109]

---

[109] With short, tight calves, the knee will bend early. But with this walk, the calves and plantar surfaces of the feet will release and lengthen, often more than from stretching, or as much as from Rolfing® SI. Additionally, even if there is a torque in the knee, it often doesn't matter because the knee is not bearing any weight in this stride. The weight is on the pivot leg, where the knee is straight. This can be the key to eliminating a runner's chronic knee problem.

Once you are doing the stride, then focus on secondary areas:

- Keep your eyes on the horizon. Train yourself to increase your peripheral vision. Learn to trust that you don't need to look down. You will see what you need to see. And because you are leaning forward, you will actually be better able to recover if you lose your balance.

- Elbows are out to your sides, not pointing behind. (Elbows rotated back promote adducting the scapulae along with rotating the shoulders back. This pulls your whole body back as your head goes forward.[110]) As you run, your thumbs should point towards each other, not up.

- Your knees are headlights—have them shine straight ahead. Everyone has some eversion of their feet. Don't be concerned where your feet go. Focus on your knees going straight.[111]

- Relax your feet. Let them flop. At first, you have to make them flop. This is the high point of the exaggeration[112]—making a flopping sound as you walk. Slap your feet on the floor. Don't

---

[110] Twenty years ago, an Olympic marathon runner came to me complaining about "weak shoulders." I assured him the problem wasn't weakness; it was tension from holding them up and rotating his arms back. Once he learned to drop his arms and his shoulders, his exercise asthma was gone.

[111] The Olympic marathon runners I had as clients had the straightest legs I have ever seen, yet they had a little eversion. Anyone I see with straight feet is working at it, torqueing their feet and ankles to create a straight or inverted foot.

[112] Not allowing the foot to land in a relaxed and natural manner tightens the foot, particularly the plantar surface. Plantar fasciitis and heel spurs develop from the fascia becoming short, thick, and brittle. Flopping the foot allows its twenty-six bones to start articulating, as well as allowing the ankle to increase its range of motion.

force them... just pretend you're a kid trying to make as much noise as you can. If you're flopping, you're leaning forward properly and you aren't lifting your foot or toes[113], which is a consequence of leaning back. Virtually everyone mistakenly holds their feet when they walk or run.[114]

- Push a cart. For my elderly clients (or anyone unsure of their balance), I encourage them to go to the supermarket and push the cart around to get the falling forward. A client, who had been a marathon runner, finally got the walk one day when she found herself running through an airport, pushing a luggage cart. She finally got what it was to fall forward.

- The forward falling momentum keeps us upright, just as a bike will stay upright once it is moving forward.

Let go:

- Use pain or discomfort as a signal to let go or remember the *Natural Walk* and Run form.

- Don't push through pain. It's telling you something. Figure out what you need to relax or fix in your form to get the pain to go away. For example:

- feels jarring – you're landing on your heels

---

[113] McDougall, op. cit., 91. There is a quote from the highly respected running coach, Dr. Joe Vigil, about the Tarahumara Indians: "Look how they point their toes down, not up."

[114] Lifting the foot causes the anterior tibialis to feel like the tibia. Eventually, many runners develop shin splints from the fascia being torn off the perioste-um of the tibia as it keeps being traumatized and thickening from the micro-traumas of a muscle doing a job it is not meant to do.

- breathing is a strain – you're holding your breath, tensing your shoulders, maybe you're hunched over, or your stomach is tense

- knees hurt – you're not leaning forward, you're lifting your toes, not letting hips and legs swing naturally, or taking too wide of a gait

- shins hurt – you aren't flopping, rather, you're lifting your feet and possibly your toes

Common Symptoms and Benefits

After years of leaning back, with the calves never exercising full range of motion, Natural Running or Walking may leave the client feeling discomfort or pulled muscles. As I tell my clients, if you went to the gym and did bicep curls by only lifting the dumbbell two inches, your bicep would shorten. That is exactly what happens to the calves; they shorten from years of never being fully extended. (In a supine position, you see that their calves pull their heels up, causing their feet to point down.) It's as if we all wore high heels for years. After a few sessions of Rolfing® SI and several weeks of practice, the calf muscles will start to lengthen.

A similar thing can occur with the plantar surface of the feet: the feet might ache as they release, particularly feet with high arches. One client gained two shoe sizes from Rolfing® SI work and from doing the walk as his feet unclenched and stretched out. Another client created a sustainable arch from developing his intrinsic muscles. Frozen joints can break loose. At first it's painful, but once released, clients become ecstatic.

This walk will take a posterior pelvis and make it horizontal, thereby creating a lumbar curve. Some people worry about that because they were told to tuck their pelvises to reduce its curve. People who never had a butt develop a butt. As the pelvis finds a balanced position, the lateral structures of the legs cease to propel the person forward and the core muscles guide the fall, cellulite will often disappear. (This will be the last thing to happen, usually from months of doing the walk.)

Sometimes clients report that their shoulders or necks hurt when they didn't before the Rolfing® SI sessions. I show them that their old posture and walk necessitated holding and explain that after the Rolfing® SI process releases the shoulders and neck, they will feel the effects of reverting to their old habits. As they master falling forward and breathing, the shoulders find a new, relaxed home. Foot releasing is less difficult; other than a frozen joint, there shouldn't be much discomfort. If there is, it's usually a sign that the person is not doing the walk correctly.

Even five minutes per day of going out and practicing the *Natural Walk* for a few weeks is usually sufficient. I encourage people to learn it by themselves and not while walking a dog or talking to a friend. Once they get it, they won't need to concentrate on it. Again, exaggeration is the key. As strange as it feels and looks, it works. It takes time to unlearn a strong unconscious movement pattern and to stretch out restrictions.[115,116] The biggest complaint I hear is that it doesn't feel natural. I say, if it felt natural, you would already be doing it. We are creating a new set point for natural—or more accurately, recreating an old, correct set point for natural.

---

[115] McDougall, op. cit., 170 on how stretching does not work.

[116] Van Mechelen, W., H. Hlobil, H.C.G. Kemper, W.J. Voorn, and H.R. de Jongh, "Prevention of running injuries by warm-up, cool-down, and stretching exercises." *Am J Sports Med*, Sept. 1993, vol. 21, no. 5, 711-719. Available at http://ajs.sagepub.com/content/21/5/711.abstract?sid=2ed54888-b116-4237-a122-7d6ba3df12d6. This study, with a follow-up study at the University of Hawaii, showed how stretching produces the same results as no stretching in terms of injury prevention. I continually see that stretching does not release the chronic fascial adhesions, and not just with runners.

Conclusion

The beauty of Natural Walking and Natural Running is its simplicity. Clients might resist the exaggerated practice form, but they all understand it and feel it. Most will practice it. Many have transformed their bodies with it. Several of my clients who never thought they could run are running races and marathons.

Many years ago, I had a client who was a business executive in his sixties. Earlier in his life, he'd been a professional athlete. In his sixties, he was still athletic and loved his daily walks. Flat feet and back pain eventually brought him to me. Being a walker, he had ample time to practice the *Natural Walk*. As a fellow flat-footed man, I knew it could be a little more challenging to master this walk with flat feet, but he was determined. Every week he would come in showing me his latest accomplishment. He was slowly getting it. About seven weeks into the series, he came in beaming like a ten-year-old boy who'd hit his first homerun. You would have thought he'd had his first orgasm after hearing him describe the first peak exercise experience of his life. That day he went for his walk and fell into a zone where time and space ceased to exist. He said he could have been out five minutes or five hours and he wouldn't have known how long it was.

You are welcome to take what I have written and use it or experiment with it. I created a free short eBook for runners that is equally applicable to walkers. Go to www.RunningFlow.com to download the eBook. Feel free to share it with your clients.

Rolfing® SI Healing Crisis - Understanding How We Get Well

Why Do I Feel Worse When I Should Be Feeling Better?

You decided to experience Rolfing® SI to feel better, and now you are feeling worse. How is this possible, you ask? For the same reason you would feel worse after starting to get back into shape. Your body is getting rid of what is preventing it from being healthy. You've progressed from addressing just the symptoms to healing the underlying causes.

After 35 years of my own healing crises and supporting thousands of clients through theirs, I began to understand that, just like remodeling an old house to achieve a higher state of order, the old order must be disturbed. Rolfing® SI does an excellent job of breaking up the old patterns that limit your vitality.

Let me affirm that you are *not* going nuts: the old or weird symptoms you feel are not imagined. I doubt they represent anything serious, and they will pass. Also, just because you go through a series of Rolfing® SI sessions you may not necessarily have a healing crisis.

The phenomenon of your body and mind detoxing and going through a healing crisis is not often talked about and it should be. Understanding this process can make a consequence of Rolfing® SI or any holistic therapy go from being scary to just an inconvenience. Explaining what is going on to hundreds of clients and students over the years made a huge difference in their experiences.

My intent in writing this is to create a larger framework which will help you understand the entire process of getting well. It is also to give you some things you can do to mitigate the downside of the process. This chapter will be longer than my usual chapters, since I have learned that when a client is experiencing a healing crisis, more information is frequently better. I have divided the article into twelve sections:

Concept

When an imbalance has existed for a while, the entire system exhausts its ability to compensate, causing sub-systems to begin to fail. Any gardener knows that the soil can only be depleted for so long before the plants start showing signs of weakness. Weak plants become vulnerable to attack and disease. Our bodies are no different. Years of stress and exposure to toxic substances weakens them.

Scientists call this adaptation to the constant stress "allostatic load."[117] It happens where a new baseline of homeostasis is created. Your body is meant to sustain a high level of output to survive; it is just not designed to do it for an extended period of time. Post-traumatic stress disorder (PTSD) is a specific illustration of exhausted coping mechanisms.

To permanently alleviate symptoms, the whole system—the entire body—needs to be released. The hyper-state, the "allostatic load" that was created to survive, must be turned off. When the body starts to come down from being wired, many of the consequences begin to be

---

[117] http://en.wikipedia.org/wiki/Allostatic_load

released. This is not much different than a person withdrawing from an addiction. Not only does the body excrete the addictive substance, but it can also release many of the other substances and emotions that were linked to the original substance.

The most common complaint that brings a client in to see me is back pain. In most cases, this person has tried other therapies that helped for a while, but inevitably, the back pain would return. In the process of seeing me, the clients often begin to realize that their back pain was tied to many other long-term conditions, such as a short leg, an old sports injury, chronic stress, or kidney toxicity. Through the course of Rolfing®, the body begins to unwind. The first feeling one has is relief—in this case, when the back becomes looser. A few more sessions frequently causes deeper structures to let go. When this occurs, the held state of chronic stress, the allostatic load, starts to release. This is when true healing occurs. It is also when a healing crisis is more likely to occur.

The disassembling of the old world order, the disruption of what was a pseudo-balance state as the prelude to creating a higher state of balance, can bring about the healing crisis. I have had many clients say they felt as if their world was falling apart. Indeed, their internal world was. This purification process restores the body's natural ability to exist in a more relaxed, adaptable, and balanced state. The shift from a body that is getting worse to one that is getting better is the *turning point,* the healing *crisis*.

Leaving Survival

We are hardwired to survive—above all else. If you were to run away from a mountain lion, you would not be aware of the nicks and bruises you incurred. Nor would your body focus its resources on healing those injuries. It would focus all of its resources on escaping. Once safe, you and your body become aware of your injuries as the immediate threat dissipates. When you release the shock and exhaustion of running for your life, the healing begins.

What makes Rolfing® SI powerful is that it pulls the plug on this "stuck" state of survival, thereby allowing healing to begin. From working with post-traumatic stress clients, I learned that the trauma needs to be released before real healing can occur. If the client remains in trauma (or post-traumatic stress), a state of survival, he or she does not have the resources to allocate to healing.

We are all, in one way or another, stuck in chronic stress or post-traumatic stress, the constant state of fight or flight wherein the autonomic nervous system's sympathetic[118] subsystem stays on. This wears us out. When Rolfing® SI releases it, all hell can break loose. The physical and emotional imbalance is upset as the energy that went to surviving goes toward healing. Often, the body first will purge the stress and/or toxins that held it in its current state, as these are what prevented it from healing. Take, for example, releasing the fascial adhesions that held stress and restricted circulation. This release can result in the physical and emotional "toxins" letting go, and thus temporarily upsetting the balance of the system as they are let go and integrated. The body has its own intelligence and sense of what is needed to optimize the healing process.

Scope

These healing crises can occur within the first few sessions of Rolfing®, or they can occur months after the basic series of sessions are completed. The healing crisis can last a few hours, in the case of something like a headache, or for months with a more sustained feeling of exhaustion.

The body may progress through cycles of contraction and expansion several times in several areas. This represents the natural process the body goes through as it heals. The body will go into aberration, which is to say that it will exaggerate its strain before it is released. In homeopathy, the worsening of a symptom is an indication that the correct reme-

---

[118] http://en.wikipedia.org/wiki/Autonomic_nervous_system

dy was used. It is as if the body was prevented from undergoing this aberration, and once allowed to experience the strain, the body can relax.

I can remember back in the mid '70s when I healed my back through Rolfing® SI. For no apparent reason, my back would start getting tight and twisted. One day it would be my low back twisting to the right. The next day my mid-back would be twisting to the left. Finally, it would finish with my neck twisting to the right on the third day..

The body also goes through cycles of building up to new plateaus of healthfulness. Then, after a period of time, the process of disruption can resume until the next plateau is reached. Often, after experiencing a new level of health, a healing crisis occurs. I know it is disconcerting to be feeling great and the next day be sick, but hang in there. Eventually, you will find a stable level.

Healing crises can repeat themselves. Everyone has their unique set of healing crises based on their stress and experiences. In the course of receiving Rolfing® SI, the first time a particular healing crisis occurs is usually the worst. As the process repeats these crises should decrease in intensity and length.

Healing crises can be identical to the symptoms you had in the past or they may be something you have never experienced. In most cases, if you had a chronic problem, even if you had not experienced it for years, it will probably manifest itself as a crisis. This re-experience is usually a holographic slice of what the condition used to be. It is not uncommon for you to encounter a reaction that you don't recall having experienced before. I have had a few of those.

What is Happening?

Now that you have a sense of why a healing crisis occurs, let's discuss what's really going on. Essentially, your body and your mind are detoxing. The simplest reason that Rolfing® SI creates this detox is because the fascia, the connective tissue that Certified Rolfers™ release, held all the toxins and stress of the body. When the fascial network begins to relax and become suppler, the circulation into once restricted areas begins to increase. The blood flushes out deposits that were locked in the soft tissue of the body including its organs.

When this occurs, it may not feel like a good thing, but trust me—it is. What was deposited in the tissue was preventing the body from functioning optimally. It is not much different than attempting to increase the flow in an old pipe. For that to happen, the gunk needs to be roto-rootered out.

The body is always processing the by-products of life, much like a sewer plant. It is when the sewer plant gets backed up that there is a problem. The liver and kidneys handling the water soluble waste can get overloaded when the blood is carrying too much of the flushed out toxins. Then when the back-up organs such as the lungs, colon, and skin can't handle the toxins, there is a healing crisis. It's not much different than when storm sewers run into the sewer system after a heavy rain, causing the sewer plant to discharge untreated effluent directly into a river.

Other holistic traditions have their explanations of what occurs during a healing crisis. Oriental medicine speaks about the five elements (the ten organs) either supporting each other or conflicting with each other. If one organ pair is not doing its job and the others can't pick up its load, the entire system becomes sick.

Homeopathy[119] tells us that the most recent symptoms will be released first and the older ones later. This means that if you injured your back three years ago and your leg 20 years ago, you are more likely to have a healing crisis that affects your back first. It is worth mentioning that I have seen—and experienced—old injuries and illnesses forgotten. I regularly ask clients if they have ever injured a certain area or had a particular illness. Because it happened in the past, and the current problems do not seem connected to these older problems, they often don't remember.

---

[119] http://en.wikipedia.org/wiki/Homeopathy

Homeopathy does a good job explaining how our normal medical treatment, allopathic medicine[120], often represses symptoms of illness and hinders the natural healing process. Consequently, when a truly holistic approach, such as homeopathy, or Rolfing® SI, impacts the body, the incomplete cycle of healing that a drug might have stopped is reactivated and, ideally, completed. In the course of treatment, layers are peeled away, much like the proverbial peeling of the onion.

Constantine Hering, M.D. (1800-1880)[121], the father of American home-opathy, observed three phenomena concerning the progression of symptoms through the course of healing:

The first progresses from the deepest part of the organism—the mental and emotional levels and the vital organs—to the external parts, such as skin and extremities. *The second* is the reversal of their original chrono-logical order of occurrence. *The third* flows from the upper to the lower parts of the body.

Old or sub-clinical (not medically observable) infections can die off. These very low-grade infections can be bacterial, viral, or fungal. A lin-gering infection may finally leave as the soft tissue of the body increases it circulation and vitality. As the infection dies off, much like with a common flu, there can be uncomfortable side effects such as fever, body aches, chills, nausea, and more.

Many years ago, I came across an article that discussed the way in which these old infections are stored in the soft tissue like a computer virus waiting to infect a computer. Receiving Rolfing® SI can be similar to running an anti-virus program. Occasionally, when these infections are taken out, they let us know they were there.

---

[120] http://en.wikipedia.org/wiki/Allopath

[121] http://www.hpathy.com/biography/c-hering.asp

It bears mentioning that Rolfing® SI breaks up old scar tissue. Scar tissue occurs when the body's fascia becomes stressed either from one specific trauma or from what I call "serial micro-traumas" from physical and/or emotional stress. Not only can this scar tissue cause many of your symptoms, it also restricts your organs' ability to function at an optimal level. The best example of the impact of fascial scar tissue restriction occurs in clients who have had colonics (professional enemas) and could not get a thorough purge. Then, after we would release their abdomen, their colonic therapist would be amazed by what came out at their next session.

Over the years, I have had a cadre of other professionals, such as holistic medical doctors, send me clients with the intent of breaking up systemic scar tissue so their treatment could work. There was one medical homeopathic physician in Phoenix who regularly sent me patients that would not respond to treatment. Usually, after a few Rolfing® SI sessions, I sent the client back to him. Once the client's body was relaxed, it was as if it went from being a brick to a sponge, able to absorb the homeopathic and herbal treatments of the other professionals. These clients' releases frequently followed a healing crisis.

Symptoms

Symptoms range from the most subtle physical release to the occasional, intense emotional release. Here is list of some of the most common healing crisis reactions I've observed in the past 35 years:

- extreme fatigue

- listlessness, feeling "spaced-out" and/or confusion

- restlessness

- emotional sensitivity

- melancholy

- neediness and/or wanting to be left alone

- outbursts of emotions such as: anger, fear/anxiety, sadness/grief

- dizziness, a feeling of spinning

- cramps and deep aches

- diarrhea and nausea

- insomnia

- cold and flu-like symptoms

- food poisoning symptoms

- fever and/or chills

- mucus discharge, sinus congestion

- frequent urination and/or urinary tract discharges

- strong body order and bad breath

- skin eruptions, such as: pimples, boils, hives, and rashes

- strange dreams

- at times may feel stronger and generally better in some ways during the healing crisis

After reading this list you may ask yourself, why would I want to experience Rolfing® SI? I assure you that it is not as bad as it may sound. Actually, I find that people do not complain about healing crises. They are much more likely to simply want to know what is happening. Most people sense that on some level they are getting better. These healing crises can be likened to what women experience when giving birth. In the midst of the delivery they may say, "I will never do this again," yet go on to have several more kids.

We have a skewed perspective on pain in this culture. We spend billions of dollars a year lessening our pain. When we are committed to restoring our health, our focus changes to doing what it takes to heal the *cause* of the pain. Athletes learn that the pain of a workout is a means to a good end. Rolfing® SI clients start to see the effects of their Rolfing® SI in the same light.

Emotions

When clients tell me what the biggest benefits to experiencing Rolfing® SI were, they usually say that it's not that the symptoms that brought them in are long gone, but rather that their emotional/stress state is much better. I was naïve as to how much stress impacted my body and its tension level, and how much my unexpressed emotions caused that tension until months after I completed my Rolfing® SI.

A trick to avoiding or lessening healing crises is to express those emotions you haven't felt or thought you couldn't express.

This connection between our emotions and our bodies isn't as "out there" as it was 30 years ago. We are beginning to understand this connection. Rolfing® SI was a crash course in embodying this understanding. Simply put, when we had emotions that we could not express as a child—getting mad at our parents is a common one—we turned that emotion into physical tension. The father of stress research, Hans Selye, M.D, in his book *The Stress of Life*[122], calls fascia the "organ of stress." It is where stress goes. It is the primary organ of the body for holding our emotions. The facial network engulfs all muscles and organs of our body. It is everywhere, just as our stress is.

As the fascial system releases, so do the old stored emotions. It is as if someone de-encrypted a hard disc that stored old data. Stored emotions held in the body still need to express what they were unable to

---

[122] http://www.amazon.com/Stress-Life-Hans-Selye/dp/0070562121

complete or express when their trigger first occurred. For example, as kids we could not tell our parents we were mad at them. Clients have described periods where they were irritated or angry at things they had not been angry at before being Rolfed.

The emotional healing crises can be the most perplexing aspect of Rolfing® SI for clients, particularly for us men. People using control as a survival strategy can initially feel a little challenged by having their emotions take over. For some, it can get intense as they travel through what I call Evolutionary Change™.[123]

I call these clients fortunate. I say this sincerely, as it will prove to be a huge gift to those who experience such a journey. It will be unlike anything they have ever experienced. At some point in this journey, you will encounter "The Dark Night of the Soul."[124] You will feel you are stepping off an edge and into the abyss. The void that you are stepping into is the completion of parts of your life, the places you have avoided—consciously or unconsciously.

This step into the void is a leap of faith. I know it may feel as though you are being pushed, but you can step back into the life you have. It will take a conscious decision to allow the process to take you over the edge. I know that it feels like you will die. Carl Jung, MD[125] would claim that your ego was dying or that its dominant control of you was dying. It does not want to lose control, and it will fight.

For the few who experience this journey, it will change your life forever. You will never be the same. Rolfing® is by no means the only way to catalyze this transformation. I have seen other therapies do this, along with spiritual ceremonies, and life crises break open this process.

---

[123] http://owenmarcus.com/deep-change/evolutionary-change/

[124] http://en.wikipedia.org/wiki/Dark_Night_of_the_Soul

[125] http://en.wikipedia.org/wiki/Carl_Jung

A special note: no matter how great you may feel after traveling through a healing crisis, allow for some time to integrate the changes into your life. Do not make any important decisions until you are rested. There are times when there may be a need to seek professional support in the form of counseling or psychotherapy if very intense or deeply-seated emotions arise. Most communities have psychotherapists that are familiar with Rolfing® SI and the body/mind connection.

Support

Now that you understand the concept of the healing crisis, you understand what is occurring and you are familiar with the symptoms. Let's discuss what you can do to support yourself through the process.

Creating a new framework for your reactions and how that can generate a healing crisis in itself can be significant. When I take a few minutes to outline what a healing crisis actually is, the client starts to relax and often gets excited about getting well. It is like some part of her knew that a good thing was happening, but there was no one supporting that belief in her world.

My first suggestion is always to surrender to the process. This does not mean suffering. It means attempting to accept that your body/mind is healing itself. We live in a society that doesn't encourage us to slow down. Allowing our body and its health to be the priority can be the most difficult aspect of a healing crisis.

You don't need to do this alone. Call your Rolfer™ or your healthcare provider if you have any questions. When the body releases, so can old held emotions, and finding a practitioner that appreciates this may be of support.

Frequently, my clients come to realize that their biggest reason for developing the symptoms that brought them to me was how tense they were from always being on the go. Their healing crises can be their bodies' attempt to rest their internal organs.

For us Type-A's, slowing down and resting is sacrilege. I have struggled with "walking my talk" of slowing down. My head can come up with all the reasons I need to do something as I continue to deny my body's voice. For those who are athletes, this can mean not training. I know athletes have many reasons why they *must* train—I have heard them all. I have also seen hundreds of clients come back and tell me that slowing down their workouts or suspending them for a period of time was the best thing they did. I had a few men come back to me after a month of not lifting to tell me they weren't weaker, and in fact, they were stronger. With a confused look on their face, they asked how that was possible. It is possible because Rolfing® SI made their structure stronger, their muscles had more circulation, and they were more relaxed.

You may prevent a healing crisis if you immediately slow down, rest, and support your body. This may mean canceling a few activities, going to bed early, not having those three beers, and relaxing.

Support Through Expressing Emotions

I discovered that if you can take what was emotional stress stored in the body and convert it back to expressed emotions, healing crises can be avoided or reduced in intensity. To facilitate this I have recommended to clients that they go out and rent a set of movies that represent the five basic emotions: fear, anger, sadness, worry, and pretense (false happiness). I have sometimes added sexual passion to the list if I believed there was some stored sexual energy. The goal here is to prime your emotional expression.

We are meant to give with our emotions and hold with our bodies, as Swift Deer, a Native American elder/shaman would say. When we can begin to give with our emotions, our bodies no longer have to do what they were not designed to do, and we begin to relax.

You can also catalyze the giving of your emotions to avoid a healing crisis by calling an old friend or lover and getting honest with him/her. If it means making amends, do it. You will feel great afterwards. Or, maybe it could involve telling this person how much he or she means to you.

For others, going into a reflective space can help. Praying, meditating, or performing a ceremony may help move you through a healing crisis. In the midst of the chaos of the crisis, you may find a calm you have never experienced. The eye of the storm can bring fabulous insights.

Reducing the ways you tax your body, and particularly your detoxing systems, will lessen the crisis. Don't give your body more than it can handle; support it with rest and good food. I have also suggested to clients that they back off on their Rolfing® SI if they are in a healing crisis. That would also hold true for other catalyzing therapies.

It can be helpful to receive therapies that support the body's elimination of the toxins and stored metabolic waste and rest—for some it may be colon therapy, for others a massage or an acupuncture treatment.

You can research blood cleansing herbs that assist the body in minimizing the effects of detoxing. Enzymes, principally systemic (proteolytic) enzymes[126] can help break up what the body is attempting to rid itself of. Fasting or eating a raw food diet might assist. My warning here is if you are run down, weak, or thin, then a fast might not be right for you. If you are considering fasting, please do some research on how to do it right.

There are activities that can support your body in detoxing in a more graceful way. Saunas and steam baths, particularly if you brush your skin, can help your skin to detox. Soaking in an Epsom salt bath can help. Lying in the sun can be rejuvenating. Yes, I know that the sun has a bad rap, but that is changing. There is more research out that is saying the sun in moderation is much better for us than once believed.

---

[126] http://www.newswithviews.com/Howenstine/james174.htm

Social and Emotional Support

Social support can be a key to reducing healing crises. Finding people or a group that understands what it is to travel the healing journey may take some work. Many "support groups" focus on an illness. These groups aren't focused on the process of getting well. I have seen instances in which a person in one of these groups who is really committed to getting well actually becomes ostracized.

Realize that getting well and addressing old issues is, unfortunately, not the norm. That said, there are people and groups that have gone through what you have gone through.

It bears mentioning that you may go through a period where you feel reclusive. That is normal. Allow it. You may also find that you are drifting away from some of your friends. This social healing crisis is a strange one. It's like discovering that what was once your favorite food is no longer your favorite food. You may find yourself less tolerant of some of your friends' behaviors. It is uncomfortable. I can say however, from my personal and professional experience, that in the long run you will have relationships that are even more enjoyable.

Here are some suggestions on where to start your communication with your friends and family to get the energy moving:

- speak about what you are going through, as best as you can tell others your experience and listen to them respond

- communicate your feelings and needs

- set your boundaries; tell others what is not okay for you. This can be the most difficult thing to do

- share with them your commitment to being well

- share with them this book

- share with them that they may experience the effect of old emotions coming out:

- I call this co-lateral damage—often old anger that was not okay to express as a child will be directed towards your spouse

- warn them that it is not about them

- you are releasing old emotions and learning that it is okay to do so

- the fact they are the target represents your trust in them. That may not be a significant consolation, but it's true

- I have always seen this work out for the best

Preventing a Healing Crisis

Anticipate that your body/mind will detox. Create a network of support using what I mentioned earlier. Be proactive with your communications and your detoxing; don't wait until you are in a position in which you have to do it.

Also, investigate detoxing programs. There are many of these programs available. They may include cleansing herbs, bulking and cleansing agents for the colon, and a whole protocol of how to use them. Using a complete program or working with a holistic health professional to supervise the program can make a difference in your overall health and the effect Rolfing® SI has on your body.

Develop your own ways to release your emotions. It may mean finding a good therapist or group that focuses on emotional maturity. To start your own group you can go to my site: Men Corps[127] to download the free protocol to start and run your own group. These micro-communities prove to be much more than the typical support group.

---

[127] http://www.mencorps.org/

Over the years of starting and training men to lead men's groups, I've seen men transform their lives to places they thought didn't exist.

My blog www.owenmarcus.com contains posts that you may find useful in supporting your larger process of change.

Others will tell you keeping your body alkaline can prevent illness. Junk food and stress make your body acidic, which allows infections and disease to fester. Again, rest and sleep are in order. You can be doing all the right things, but if you are not resting, you can't rejuvenate.

Conclusion

From many of my own healing crises and thousands of Rolfing® SI clients, along with clients in other settings, I can say that no matter how intense a healing crisis is, it will pass. If you or any friend of yours has any concern about what is occurring, seek medical advice.

As strange as this may sound, enjoy the healing crisis as much as you can. It is your gift to your body to help it get well. Avoid turning from one who thinks this is all New Age hyperbole to the fanatic on a constant cycle of purging him or herself. Allow your body to travel its own path; your job is to support it.

Your body has an amazing ability to heal itself. Deep within, it knows how to do its job to break up what is preventing that natural process of healing, and then support it once it starts. As a Certified Rolfer™, I don't see myself as a healer, I see myself as the instigator who stirs up things so you and your Creator can do the healing. This healing energy is what will renew your body and keep you young.

The process of experiencing a healing *crisis* becomes a process of where you begin to see yourself being in a defining moment—where on some level you are committing to a new depth of wellness. The crisis evolves to be a portal where you step through to a new place of health. Once on the other side, not only are you different, you do not want to go back.

I strongly encourage you to speak to your Certified Rolfer™ about your feelings and experiences; he or she can be a great resource along with other local providers. Use this book as an adjunct resource to assist you in your Rolfing® SI and healing journey. I wish you the best on this journey.

None of this would have been possible without all my Rolfing® SI clients. These people trusted me to help them. They allowed me to lean my elbow into their soft tissue. Then they came back for another session—and sent their friends and family!

Before I ever touched a client, I saw a Certified Rolfer™. Jason Kayne, my first Certified Rolfer™, immediately inspired me with the results he created from my first session. After that one session, I was hooked. Before there was Jason, there was Ida Rolf, PhD. Dr. Rolf saw what was missing, created a therapy to fill that gap, and never gave up putting it out to the public.

The editing of much of the content was originally done by my good friend, client, and champion Theresa Renner. She continues to turn my dyslexic words into readable prose. Stacy Jenkins, another good friend also edited this book. I should have had them in high school when I was flunking English.

The help of Certified Rolfer™ Chris Hayden and Gibney Siemion in proofing the book is greatly appreciated by all of us. Jim Ryan did the final polish of the manuscript proving that there is always more to be done.

Finally, I want to thank you, the reader, for investing in the book—and in me—to provide you with what you want from your body and Rolfing SI. I encourage you to go to my Rolfing SI site, and signed up for our mailing list: www.align.org/mailing.

Owen Marcus, MA
Certified Advanced Rolfer™
219 Cedar Street, Suite A
Sandpoint, ID 83864
www.align.org

Stay Informed

Go to www.align.org/book to sign up for our email list.

Disclaimer

Your Mileage May Vary

In 30+ years of Rolfing® thousands of clients, I have learned a lot about what Rolfing® can and can't do. I have attempted to use my experience with Rolfing® to assist you in determining if it would be appropriate for you. It is not for everyone; but please use this book as a guide to determine if it is right for you.

Rolfing® Structural Integration is not involved with the treatment of disease, illness, or disorders of any kind, nor does it substitute for medical diagnosis or treatment when such attention is needed. Likewise, the Certified Rolfer™ does not diagnose or treat any illness, disease, or other physical or mental disorder of the person, and nothing said or done by the Instructor should be misconstrued as such. Any relief of physical or emotional symptoms is coincidental to the Rolfing® SI process and is not a goal of Rolfing® SI.

Consult your own physician or licensed healthcare practitioner regarding the applicability of any opinions or recommendations with respect to your symptoms or medical/psychological condition. Information shared in this book or personally is shared for educational purposes.

This information is not to be used to diagnose, treat, cure, or prevent a disease. Owen Marcus is not a medical doctor. Rolfing® does not replace conventional medicine, but can be a useful supplement to medical treatment.

Rolfing® designates the Rolf Institute's brand of structural integration, the discipline developed by the late Ida P. Rolf, PhD. While the Rolf Institute is Dr. Rolf's original school of structural integration, it is now one of many schools of structural integration. Rolfing® Structural Integration designates the practice of structural integration by graduate members of the Rolf Institute, who are licensed to use its service marks.

Rolfing® is owned by the Rolf Institute

Rolfing®, Rolfers™, and Rolf Movement Practitioners™ are all registered trademarks owned by the Rolf Institute.

Owen Marcus

In 1980, Owen Marcus opened up his new Rolfing® (SI) practice in Scottsdale, AZ. The practice quickly evolved to a holistic medical clinic employing other Rolfers™, physicians, nutritionists, massage therapists and additional providers. They contracted research with Arizona State University on how Rolfing® SI improved athletic performance. Owen regularly treated professional and Olympic athletes. He also designed and taught professional development courses for the Rolf Institute.

He continues to share innovative techniques with his colleagues as well with his clients. Owen's articles explain how holistic therapies can be woven together to create amazing change. His story of how he healed his Asperger's Syndrome, dyslexia and dyspraxia evolved from his inspiration to his unique understanding of how healing works.

Today he lives in Sandpoint, ID where he writes and teaches on men's and relationship issues. His blog www.owenmarcus.com is a leader in the field of men's issues. Free to Win, www.freetowin.CO is Owen's training company. They offer men mentoring, two day men's group trainings, and virtual products to help men be free to live their own lives.

His Rolfing® SI site, www.align.org continues to be ranked as the top Rolfers site under the term Rolfing® SI because it's an excellent resource for the public.

Index

A

abdomen, 43, 44, 45, 46, 47, 49, 62, 63, 115, 117, 152

accident, 17, 40, 41

Achilles Tendon, 84

acupuncture, 6, 8, 19, 26, 40, 44, 59, 104, 158

acute, 3, 6, 8, 37, 40, 41, 62, 70, 124

adrenalin, 113

aging, 12, 20, 78, 83, 94, 95, 96, 98, 103, 117, 119, 125, 126

align, 8

allergies, 127

allopathic medicine, 18, 71, 151

allostatic load, 146, 147

alternative therapies, 38, 76

Andrew Weil, MD, 18, 54, 58

anger, 153, 157, 160

ankylosing spondylitis, 127

anti-inflammatories, 86

anti-inflammatory drugs, 33, 48

Arizona, 25, 29, 33, 42, 71, 82, 90, 112, 129, 131, 137, 165

Arizona State University, 33, 82, 90, 131, 165

arthritis, 39, 126, 127, 128

Asperger's Syndrome, 76, 165

athletes, 4, 17, 34, 69, 79, 90, 118, 119, 157, 165

Auburn University, 29

auto accident, 40

auto accidents, 37

autoimmune disorders, 127

awareness, 3, 11, 64, 72, 78, 97, 107, 132

B

back pain, 18, 34, 47, 60, 61, 62, 64, 66, 70, 89, 92, 93, 101, 105, 110, 144, 147

balance, 8, 30, 37, 42, 69, 93, 98, 99, 104, 140, 141, 147, 148

barefoot, 23, 24, 29, 30, 130, 135, 136

baseball pitchers, 20, 52

bed, 34, 35, 36, 61, 113, 114, 115, 116, 157

Benno M. Nigg, 23

biochemical, 73

biometrically, 129

Birkenstocks, 29

Body by Science, 81

bones, 3, 22, 23, 26, 27, 31, 36, 38, 47, 50, 64, 65, 80, 96, 97, 105, 109, 110, 140

Born to Run, 136

breathing, 28, 37, 47, 64, 65, 84, 104, 105, 107, 111, 114, 122, 124, 128, 132, 133, 135, 142, 143

bunions, 21

bursitis, 50

C

cancer, 8, 102, 124

candidiasis, 127

Carl Jung, MD, 155

cartilage, 26, 31, 88, 126, 127

4 $3\frac{1}{2}$ $3\frac{1}{3}$ - 4 $3\frac{1}{2}$ $5\frac{1}{2}$ ᴌ

$$\frac{18}{3}\frac{12.5}{0.5}$$

13415 Fort Road Ed.

9 780988 703513